T0175842

Neurological Physiotherapy Pocketbook

SECOND EDITION

Edited by

Sheila Lennon, PhD, MSc, BSc, FCSP
Professor of Physiotherapy
College of Nursing and Health Sciences
Flinders University of South Australia
Adelaide, AUS

Gita Ramdharry, BSc(Hons) PG Cert, MSc, PhD
Associate Professor
Faculty of Health, Social Care and Education
Kingston University & St George's University of London
London, UK

Consultant Allied Health Professional
Queen Square Centre for Neuromuscular Diseases
The National Hospital for Neurology and Neurosurgery
University College London NHS Foundation Trust
London, UK

Geert Verheyden, PhD
Associate Professor
Department of Rehabilitation Sciences
KU Leuven - University of Leuven
Leuven, BEL

ELSEVIER

ELSEVIER

© 2018 Elsevier Limited. All rights reserved.

First edition 2009
Second edition 2018

ISBN 978-0-7020-5508-9

British Library Cataloguing in Publication Data
A catalogue record for this book is available from the British Library

Library of Congress Cataloging in Publication Data
A catalog record for this book is available from the Library of Congress

your source for books,
journals and multimedia
in the health sciences

www.elsevierhealth.com

  Working together
to grow libraries in
developing countries

www.elsevier.com • www.bookaid.org

The
Publisher's
policy is to use
**paper manufactured
from sustainable forests**

Content Strategist: *Poppy Garraway*
Content Development Specialist: *Veronika Watkins*
Project Manager: *Nayagi Athmanathan*
Designer: *Amy Buxton*
Illustration Manager: *Amy Faith Heyden*

Printed in India

Last digit is the print number: 9 8 7 6 5 4 3

CONTENTS

This *Neurological Physiotherapy Pocketbook* is intended to provide both students and qualified physiotherapists with an overview of the physiotherapy management of people with neurological conditions. This second edition has been completely revised by internationally renowned clinicians and researchers led by a new editorial team. We have also concurrently edited the fourth edition of the *Physical Management for Neurological Conditions*, which complements this pocketbook.

This pocketbook of essential facts is organised in two sections starting with seven chapters related to essential background knowledge, followed by six chapters on the most common neurological conditions encountered by physiotherapists. We hope this pocketbook continues to provide quick and easy access to essential clinical information for physiotherapists working in neurological clinical practice.

Sheila Lennon
Adelaide, Australia

Gita Ramdharry
London, United Kingdom

Geert Verheyden
Leuven, Belgium

We the editors have all worked at some point in the United Kingdom and shared ideas at many international conferences. It truly has been such an easy and collegiate experience to collaborate as editors on this pocketbook despite our widespread locations and different time zones. Fitting it into our busy clinical, academic, research and administrative workloads has been rather more challenging!

Thanks to all the students, clinicians and academic colleagues who have provided invaluable feedback on this new edition. We thank the team at Elsevier for keeping us on track in such a supportive way, with special thanks to our content editor, Veronika Watkins.

We are indebted to all our authors for generously sharing their knowledge and expertise. Last but not least, thanks to the patients who have informed our own practice.

Sheila Lennon
Adelaide, Australia

Gita Ramdharry
London, United Kingdom

Geert Verheyden
Leuven, Belgium

Clare Bassile, PT, EdD
Assistant Professor of Rehabilitation & Regenerative Medicine
Program in Physical Therapy
Columbia University Medical Center
New York, NY, USA

Adrian Capp, MSc in Adult Critical Care, BHSc Physiotherapy
Head of Therapy Services
The National Hospital for Neurology and Neurosurgery
University College London NHS Foundation Trust
London, UK

Aisling Carr, MRCP Neurol. PhD
Consultant Neurologist
Queen Square Centre for Neuromuscular Diseases
The National Hospital for Neurology and Neurosurgery
University College London NHS Foundation Trust
London, UK

Jennifer Freeman, BAppSci (Physiotherapy), PhD
Professor in Physiotherapy and Rehabilitation
Faculty of Health and Human Sciences
School of Health Professions
Plymouth University
Plymouth, UK

Jill Garner, Grad Dip Phys, Master of Clinical Rehabilitation
Lecturer in Physiotherapy
College of Nursing and Health Sciences
Flinders University of South Australia
Adelaide, AUS

Advanced Clinician in Neurorehabilitation
Rehabilitation, Aged Care and Palliative Care (RAP)
Flinders Medical Centre
Adelaide, AUS

Mariella Graziano, BSc(Hons)
Neuro – Physiotherapy Practice
16, rue Boltgen L-4038 Esch-sur-Alzette, LUX

Hilary Gunn, PhD, MSc, Grad Dip Phys
Lecturer in Physiotherapy
Faculty of Health and Human Sciences
School of Health Professions
Plymouth University
Plymouth, UK

Benita Hexter, BSc(Hons)
Clinical Specialist and Lead Physiotherapist
London Spinal Cord Injury Centre
The Royal National Orthopaedic Hospital NHS Trust
Stanmore, UK

Honorary Clinical Teaching Fellow
University College
London, UK

Brenton Hordacre, PhD, BPhty
Body in Mind Research Group
School of Health Sciences
Division of Health Sciences
The University of South Australia
Adelaide, AUS

Sheila Lennon, PhD, MSc, BSc, FCSP
Professor of Physiotherapy
College of Nursing and Health Sciences
Flinders University of South Australia
Adelaide, AUS

Alana McCambridge, PhD
Clinical Neurostimulation Lab
Graduate School of Health
Discipline of Physiotherapy
University of Technology Sydney
Sydney, AUS

James McLoughlin, BAppSc, MSc, PhD
Associate Professor
Clinical Rehabilitation
College of Nursing and Health Sciences
Flinders University of South Australia
Adelaide, AUS

Director Advanced Neuro Rehab
Payneham
Adelaide, AUS

Sue Paddison, Grad Dip Phys
Clinical Specialist and Lead Physiotherapist
London Spinal Cord Injury Centre
Royal National Orthopaedic Hospital Trust
Stanmore, Middlesex, UK

Honorary Clinical Teaching Fellow
University College London

Louise Platt, MSc in Advanced Neurophysiotherapy, BSc(Hons) Physiotherapy, BA(Hons) Business Studies
Therapy Team Lead in Neurosurgery
Therapy and Rehabilitation Services
The National Hospital for Neurology and Neurosurgery
University College London NHS Foundation Trust
London, UK

Bhanu Ramaswamy, OBE, FCSP, DProf, MSc, Grad Dip Physiotherapy
Faculty of Health and Wellbeing
Sheffield Hallam University
Sheffield, UK

Gita Ramdharry, BSc(Hons) PG Cert, MSc, PhD
Associate Professor
Faculty of Health, Social Care and Education
Kingston University & St George's University of London
London, UK

Consultant Allied Health Professional for Neuromuscular Diseases
Queen Square Centre for Neuromuscular Diseases
The National Hospital for Neurology and Neurosurgery
University College London NHS Foundation Trust
London, UK

Mark Slee, BAppSc, BMBS, FRACP, PhD
Associate Professor
Neurology
College of Medicine and Public Health
Flinders University of South Australia
Adelaide, AUS

Janne Veerbeek, PhD
Post Doctoral Physical Therapist
Department of Neurology
University of Zurich/University Hospital Zurich
Zurich, CH

Geert Verheyden, PhD
Associate Professor
Department of Rehabilitation Sciences
KU Leuven - University of Leuven
Leuven, BEL

Gavin Williams, PhD, Grad Dip, B App Sci, FACP
Associate Professor Physiotherapy Research
Physiotherapy
Epworth Healthcare
Melbourne, AUS

Department of Physiotherapy
Faculty of Medicine, Dentistry and Health Sciences
University of Melbourne
Melbourne, AUS

BACKGROUND KNOWLEDGE

CHAPTER 1

Guiding principles in neurological rehabilitation

Sheila Lennon and Clare Bassile

INTRODUCTION

Neurological rehabilitation is a process that assists individuals who experience disability to achieve and maintain optimal function and health in interaction with their environment (WHO 2001). It requires an active partnership between the patient, their family and a team of health and social care professionals.

The role of the physiotherapist working in neurology is to help the patient experience and relearn optimal movement and functional activity. Movement re-education and the practice of functional activity are two essential components of neurological physiotherapy.

Physiotherapists use the process of clinical reasoning combined with current evidence and the patient and carer's perspective to assess, develop and evaluate an appropriate plan of care for each patient (Fig. 1.1). Assessment is always the starting point for clinical reasoning (see Chapter 4). This assessment process is used to guide intervention by identifying clinical problems. The rehabilitation team together with patient and his or her family collaboratively agree on joint treatment goals before devising a treatment plan composed of interventions that should be based on the best available evidence. Standardised outcome measures with published reliability, validity and sensitivity should be used to establish a baseline of performance before rehabilitation, then at key strategic points to document change as a result of interventions.

NEUROLOGICAL TREATMENT APPROACHES

Historically the content, structure and aims of physical therapies have been based on therapist preference for a specific treatment approach, such as the Bobath concept. A Cochrane review by Pollock et al (2014) has reiterated that physical rehabilitation should not be limited to named approaches, but rather should be composed of evidence-based physical techniques, regardless of historical or philosophical origin. Thus components selected within therapy sessions should be

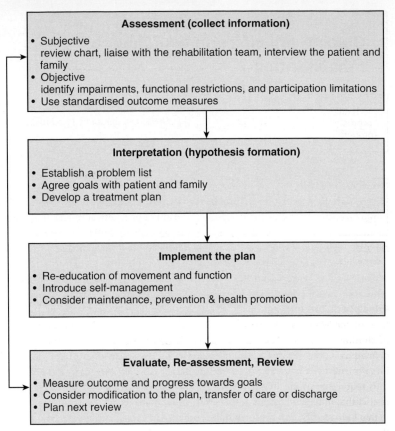

Fig. 1.1
Clinical reasoning in neurological rehabilitation (Garner and Lennon 2018 with permission).

evidence based rather than based on therapist preference for a specific treatment approach (Kollen et al 2009).

A CONCEPTUAL FRAMEWORK FOR NEUROLOGICAL REHABILITATION

A conceptual framework composed of 10 guiding principles is essential to enable physiotherapists to determine their assessment and intervention strategies (Fig. 1.2).

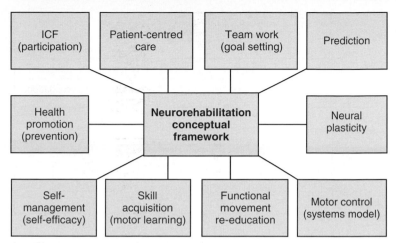

Fig. 1.2
A conceptual framework for neurological rehabilitation.

Principle 1: The International Classification of Functioning (ICF)
In 2001 the World Health Organization (WHO) developed the ICF with the aim of shifting the focus from disability and impairments to health. Impairment is defined as a deficit in body structure or function. After a stroke, an example of impairment would be weakness leading to a limitation in the activity of walking, thus requiring the use of a wheelchair for mobility. Being in a wheelchair may restrict that individual from resuming his or her job, a limitation in participating in that individual's previous role in society. Environmental and personal factors are the contextual factors that enable the rehabilitation team to identify facilitators and barriers for the rehabilitation process, such as having a house that is wheelchair accessible without stairs (Fig. 1.3).

The ICF:
- Neurological physiotherapy should target impairments, activity and participation within the ICF (WHO 2001).
- Always link the patient's impairments to activity limitations to direct a targeted approach to the re-education of movement, function and participation.
- Changes at the level of impairment and activity are only really meaningful for the patient and the family carer if they enable them to participate in their family and community life by resuming their desired life roles, albeit in a different way.

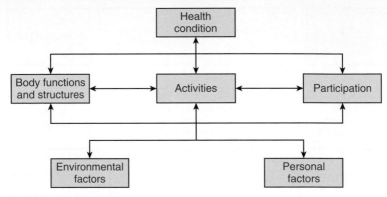

Fig. 1.3
The ICF (WHO 2001).

Principle 2: Team Work

● Is about sharing information and collaborating in goal setting, care planning and decision making. The evidence on which model of team working works best is unclear (Clarke & Forster 2015).

● Is an essential factor in improving patient outcomes. For example, patients who receive organised stroke unit care are more likely to survive their stroke, return home and become independent in looking after themselves (Stroke Unit Trialists' Collaboration [SUTC, 2013]).

● Establishing team goals helps to motivate the team and the patient, coordinate activities and ensure that all important goals are identified (Wade 2009).

● One way of facilitating appropriate goal planning is to use the SMART acronym which recommends that goals should be specific, measurable, achievable/ambitious, relevant and timed (Playford et al 2009; see Bovend'Eerdt et al 2009 for some practical guidance on how to set SMART goals).

Principle 3: Person-Centred Care

Person-centred care can be defined as a philosophy of care that encourages and supports patients and their carers to develop the knowledge, skills and confidence they need to effectively manage and make decisions about health (Health Foundation 2014; see characteristics in Box 1.1).

Carer support and involvement

Caring for people with neurological conditions can be challenging; the health care team needs to also focus on the health and well-being of the carer to reduce caregiver burden and burnout (Krishnan et al 2017). Getting involved with voluntary organisations and peer and caregiver support groups can also reduce feelings of

Box 1.1 Characteristics of person-centred practice (Whalley Hammell 2009 with permission)

- Respect for clients' values, priorities and perspectives
- Respect for clients' autonomy and right to choose and enact choices
- Seeks to realign and equalise power between therapist and client
- Provides client-oriented information to enable informed choices
- Enables clients to identify their priorities, needs and goals
- Facilitates client participation in the rehabilitation process
- Strives for collaboration and partnership in achieving client's goals
- Individualises service delivery
- Assesses the achievement of outcomes that matter to the client
- Focuses on ensuring that service provision is useful and relevant

isolation and provide additional support. Key strategies to help relieve caregiver stress and burden are (Krishnan et al 2017):

- education;
- effective communication;
- maintaining physical and psychological well-being; and
- building a local support system.

The personal experience of Fuller (2016), who cared for her husband after a devastating stroke at age 50 years for 21 years, sends some strong messages on understanding the carer experience to help the patient live as full a life as possible (see Table 1.1).

Table 1.1 Key messages from a carer on the rehabilitation process (Fuller 2017 personal communication)

Overwhelming disbelief, shock and grief	● Give the patient time to absorb that they have suffered a life-threatening illness.
Fear of the unknown, depression	● Evoke negative thoughts – is the effort worthwhile?
Take into consideration the extent of the stroke, the hidden disabilities: aphasia/dysphasia and dyspraxia	● Language barriers may impede the process of understanding a directive.
Chronic fatigue	● Inhibits clients ability to work at their full capacity.
Medication and side effects may play a negative role	● Affects comprehension.
Changes regarding rehabilitation centres: closures/reallocation	● Client having to travel longer distances to access therapy, causing disorientation – intensifies fatigue and/or anxiety.

(continued)

Table 1.1 Key messages from a carer on the rehabilitation process (Fuller 2017 personal communication)—cont'd

Limited parking or car parks situated some distance from the venue.	● Difficult for carers and clients requiring the use of wheelchairs – increases anxiety.
Don't discourage, give the client the chance to prove himself or herself	● They all want to improve – they want to be the best they can be.
Give encouragement, even if the session is a non-event	● Some will do better than others – there may be an underlying issue.
Listen to the client and/or carer	● They may have experienced/witnessed some significant gain.
Introduce achievable hobbies	● All work and no play is not a good balance.
Never, ever rule out **HOPE**	● For some, hope is the only 'positive' they can aim toward to create a change in their life. ● Hope supports adjustment, perseverance and positive outcomes; it can reflect expectations, goals and optimism, as well as act as a motivator and source of strength (Bright et al 2011).

Principle 4: Prediction

Evidence-based practice requires therapists to know and utilise the prediction literature to influence their assessments and interventions. Prediction of outcomes will lead to clearer patient expectations and better selection of interventions (Kimberley et al 2017). Prediction is never 100% accurate, and there will always be those patients who defy the odds. However, having knowledge of the prediction literature allows the therapist to:

● be realistic with the patient and carer;
● express optimism to those patients who exhibit the positive predictors; and
● promote the exhibition of these motor responses and thereby enhance recovery.

Principle 5: Neural Plasticity

Although there is always a degree of spontaneous recovery after brain damage, advances in neuroimaging have confirmed that plasticity (defined as enduring changes in structure and function) does occur after damage to the nervous system, also as a result of experience and therapy. Thus cortical maps can be modified by a variety of inputs such as sensory inputs, experience, learning and therapy, as well as in response to injury (Nudo 2013). Rehabilitation is likely to be most effective when principles of neuroplasticity are considered (see principles in Box 1.2).

Box 1.2 Principles of Neuroplasticity for Clinicians (from Hordacre & McCambridge 2018 with Permission)

- Neuroplasticity is use dependent and specific.
- Repetition and greater intensity induce neural changes.
- Neuroplasticity is time sensitive; early intervention might be better.
- Neuroplasticity is influenced by salience, motivation, feedback and attention.
- Neuroplasticity is strongly influenced by features of the environment. Enhanced sensory, cognitive, motor and social stimulation facilitate increased neuroplasticity and learning (Nithianantharajah & Hannan 2006).
- Neuroplasticity is influenced by patient characteristics such as age, genetics and stress levels.
- Adjunct therapies prime the motor system to facilitate greater neuroplastic response (Ackerley et al 2014; Byblow et al 2012).
- Pharmacology influences neuroplasticity.

What Type of Training Drives Neural Plasticity and Recovery of Function?

- Task-specific training facilitates functional as well as neural plasticity (Dimyan & Cohen 2011; Dobkin et al 2004; Hubbard et al 2009).
- Aerobic exercise enhances neural plasticity by increasing blood flow to the brain, facilitating the release of neurotrophic factors and improving brain health (brain volume). A variety of individuals with neurological diseases have been shown to lack aerobic conditioning either as a result of their impairments interfering in physical activity or adoption of a sedentary lifestyle (Brazzelli et al 2012).
- Enhancement and diminution of neural activation within the brain are dependent on the stage of skill acquisition (Dayan & Cohen 2011).
- Although evidence to date in humans is limited, animal studies suggest that there may be a critical time period for rehabilitation after stroke, with early intervention determining greater functional gains (McDonnell et al 2015).

Principle 6: Motor Control: A Systems Model

Motor control is an area of science exploring how the nervous system interacts with other body parts and the environment to produce purposeful, coordinated actions (Muratori et al 2013); thus it is critical for therapists involved in neurorehabilitation to understand how different systems within the nervous system interact to produce movement and perform tasks (see Chapter 2). For example, when a patient is learning to dress himself, he must use the movement he can reproduce in terms of his available range, strength, pain level, etc., as well as his cognitive ability to plan the task alongside external factors in the environment, e.g. bed height to perform the functional task.

A patient's actions are a consequence of (Shumway-Cook & Woollacott 2017, p. 4):
- the impairments caused by the damage;
- the compensatory strategies that enable function to be achieved in the presence of impairments;
- the effects of the environment the person has been experiencing since the lesion; and
- the person's confidence in their ability to achieve success.

Therapists aim to structure the environment or the task in a way that enables the patient to elicit or practice both the desired movement and the tasks required to achieve their goals.

Principle 7: Functional Movement Re-Education

Normative data for everyday activities help therapists to understand motor performance and the impact of impairments on these everyday activities (Carr & Shepherd 2006). Therapists place an emphasis on training control of muscles and promoting learning of relevant actions and tasks.

One of the key roles of the therapist working in neurology is to help the patient experience and relearn optimal movement and function in everyday life within the constraints imposed by the disease process and presenting impairments. Therapists are not only interested in which functional activities patients can or cannot perform, but also in how the patient moves (the quality of movement) to execute these activities. It is always preferable to prioritise the practice of functional activities selected in collaboration with the patient; however, if the patient has impairments that make it difficult to practice these tasks directly, therapists may also need to address impairments or practice specific movements either before or during a modified version of functional task practice. For example, a patient may not have any signs of motor activity in the lower limb to practice the task of walking. In this case, the patient may require either hands-on assistance from therapists or support from assistive technologies, e.g. a partial body weight support system in order to practice the task of walking or may have to practice activation of muscles in a gravity neutral environment prior to voluntary activation during walking.

The aims of neurological physiotherapy can be summed up using the acronym RAMP for recovery, adaptation, maintenance and prevention (Fig. 1.4). There are different stages in patient management where these aims may have different priorities. Understanding the nature of the pathology and the prognosis for recovery in collaboration with patients and caregivers to establish desired goals will help determine which of these aims should be emphasised in physical interventions.

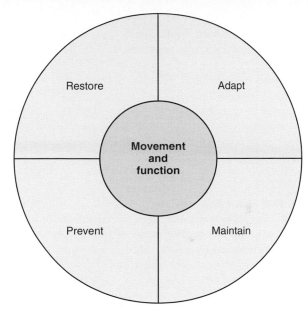

Fig. 1.4
Aims of neurological physiotherapy—RAMP.

Recovery
- Therapists ideally aim to restore movement and function in people with neurological pathology, but this may not always be possible.
- Interventions aimed at recovery of function need to be emphasised over compensation if the patient has the potential to change.

Adaptation (Compensation)
- The use of alternative movement strategies to complete a task – in other words, performing an old movement in a new way (Levin et al 2009).
- Therapists focus on promoting compensatory strategies that are necessary for function and discouraging those that may be detrimental to the patient, e.g. promoting musculoskeletal damage such as knee hyperextension (Levin et al 2009).

Maintenance
- Should be viewed as a positive achievement. Several reviews have now confirmed that functional ability can be maintained despite deteriorating impairments in progressive neurological disease (Keus et al 2014).

Prevention

- Therapy also aims to prevent the development of complications. Some common secondary complications in neurology are:
  - contractures;
  - pressure sores;
  - deep vein thrombosis;
  - pneumonia;
  - disuse atrophy;
  - deconditioning from lack of physical activity and sedentary behaviour; and
  - autonomic nervous system deregulation, e.g. fluctuations in heart rate or blood pressure.

Principle 8: Skill Acquisition

Evidence from motor learning and skill acquisition can provide some guiding principles about how to structure practice within therapy sessions to improve these aspects of skilled performance (Muratori et al 2013; Winstein et al 2014). Some tips for structuring therapy sessions are outlined in Table 1.2.

Table 1.2 Key motor learning variables for neurological rehabilitation

Key variables	Issues to consider (adapted mainly from Muratori et al 2013; Winstein et al 2014; Wulf & Lethwaithe 2016)
Practice	<ul><li>Amount (intensity or dose) (Kwakkel 2006; Lang et al 2015)</li><li>Frequency (number of repetitions)</li><li>Duration (number of minutes per session)</li><li>Variety (alter regulatory features) (Gentile 2000), e.g. transfers from different height chairs and different surface types; practicing a variety of walking tasks (ramps, obstacles, different surfaces, directions) Hornby et al 2011.</li><li>Practice schedule (e.g. blocked practice, such as five reps at each seat height) versus random practice (e.g. different seat heights each time) (Murtori et al 2013).</li><li>The practice schedule depends on a number of patient-centred issues such as experience, age, memory and task. However, there are insufficient data on which sequence works best for which patient (Muratori et al 2013; Wulf & Lethwaithe 2016).</li></ul>
Specificity of training	<ul><li>Functional task practice must be both task and context specific; therefore whenever possible practice the task (Kwakkel et al 2004; Verbeek et al 2014).</li><li>Consider critical requirements for each task (Carr & Shepherd 2003), as well as the impairments being targeted (Muratori et al 2013; Winstein et al 2014).</li></ul>

Table 1.2 Key motor learning variables for neurological rehabilitation—cont'd

Transfer of training (generalisability)	● Impairment-focused training such as strength, range, symmetry, postural sway may improve the parameters being trained, but these changes do not generalise to the activity or participation level (Kwakkel et al 2004; Muratori et al 2013; Verbeek et al 2014). ● Consider two types of transfer of training (Winstein 1991): (1) part task training: break the task down into simple steps, then put the steps back together again by practising the whole task; (2) adaptive training: simplify the task by controlling a particularly difficult part, e.g. using a body weight support system that gradually adds the body weight into gait. ● Task-related practice: some transferability will occur to a task which incorporates the components of transferring the centre of mass from the trunk to the lower extremities, e.g. practice of reaching greater than arm's length in sitting transfers to the sit-to-stand transitional activity (Dean & Shepherd 1997; Dean, Richards & Malouin 2000).
Feedback	● Frequency (How often? All or some of the time?). Do not give feedback on every trial (Muratori et al 2013; Winstein et al 1994). ● Timing (when to deliver the info: before, during or after) ● Delivery mode (visual, verbal, manual) ● Consider using extrinsic feedback or feedback with an external focus (van Vliet & Wulf 2006; Wulf 2013); e.g. for a sit-to-stand task, the focus should be on 'pushing into the floor', rather than 'push your feet into the floor', or 'stand tall' rather than 'straighten your spine/back'.
Modelling	● Demonstrate what you want the patient to do. ● Consider delivery mode, e.g. live versus videotaped versus written instruction (Laguna 2000; Reo & Mercer 2004; Williams & Hodges 2004, pp. 145–174).
Mental practice	● Defined as the act of repeating imagined movements several times with the intention of improving motor performance (Jackson et al 2001). An adjunct to physical practice; it is not better than physical practice (Braun et al 2006). ● Consider when to use it, e.g. when patient needs additional personnel to set up environment for independent practice, during rest periods or when patient is not safe to practice independently. ● Reference point for imaging—'seeing' themselves or 'feeling' themselves (Nilsen et al 2010).

● Motor skill learning can be divided into three phases: an early cognitive phase, an intermediate associative phase and an autonomous phase (Fitts & Posner 1967, cited in Schmidt & Lee 2013).
● When subjects are in the initial stage of learning, individuals should be encouraged to actively explore the environment through trial and error.

- In the later stage of skill acquisition, the focus switches from 'what to do' to 'how to do' the movement better (Schmidt & Lee 2013).
- Certain types of feedback may be beneficial at different points in skill acquisition. For example, manual guidance should mainly be used at the early cognitive stage of motor learning, especially when safety is a concern, to give the patient the idea of the movement or to control a degree of freedom.
- During the later associative and autonomous stages of skill acquisition, it is preferable for the learner to actively problem solve without relying on the therapist for feedback (Schmidt & Lee 2013; Sidaway et al 2008).
- Prescribing the most appropriate dose of practice for individual patients is a challenge because minimal data are available and a large number of factors are unknown (Lang et al 2015).
- Current best practice suggests that a minimum of 300 to 400 repetitions of actions or tasks are required per session to demonstrate gains (Birkenmeier et al 2010). For example, a minimum of 20 minutes walking practice duration over 12 sessions has been reported to improve gait in stroke survivors (Peurala et al 2014).
- Cues should be as external from the person as possible, rather than an internal focus on body movements (Wulf 2013). The movement patterns which emerge from using an external focus have been shown to be smoother, more coordinated and success achieved earlier when compared with those using an internal focus.
- To enhance the learner's expectation and increase their confidence level, the therapist must find ways which reinforce the learner's ability to achieve success. By providing positive feedback, confidence levels are increased, thereby creating the learner's expectation that he or she will achieve success (self-efficacy). Ways to enact this in the clinic are:
  - provide feedback after good trials, e.g. 'That was a good one', 'Do that again';
  - reduce perceived task difficulty: define success liberally so the criterion for a successful performance is not too difficult;
  - alleviate the learner's concerns; and
  - when using self-modelling, show their best performance.

Principle 9: Self-Management (Self-efficacy)

A recent report by NHS England (2016) defines self-management as 'any form of formal education or training for people with long-term conditions that focuses on helping people to develop the knowledge, skills and confidence to manage their own health and care effectively'. The key components involved in effective self-management are outlined in Table 1.3 (Jones & Kulnik 2018).

Table 1.3 Key components of self-management (Jones & Kulnik 2018 with permission)

Problem solving by the patient	• Deciding on the problem • Breaking it down into small steps • Thinking of various solutions • Selecting a course of action • Trying out the action or strategy • Evaluating success • Choosing an alternative action if necessary
Target or goal setting	• Translating thoughts into actions • Providing mastery experiences
Resource utilisation	• Accessing local self-help groups • Seeking expert advice • Using friends or family for support
Collaboration	• Working together with a health care professional • Sharing expertise

Self-efficacy is defined as people's beliefs about their capabilities to influence key events that affect their lives (Bandura 1997). People with a strong sense of efficacy set themselves challenging goals and maintain strong commitment to them; they continue to sustain their efforts in the face of failure or setbacks (Bandura 1997). A review specific to physiotherapy by Barron et al (2007) has shown that self-efficacy can be related to better health, higher achievement, more social integration and higher motivation to act.

Health professionals need to consider how they can promote self-efficacy and enhance their patients' self-management skills. Tailoring self-management support requires an appreciation of factors that act as barriers to or enablers of behaviour change. Two systematic reviews have found that self-management programmes improve quality of life and self-efficacy for stroke survivors in the community, but further research is required to identify key features of effective programmes (Fryer et al 2016; Lennon et al 2013).

Principle 10: Health Promotion

Promoting health is of critical importance to the field of neurological rehabilitation. The WHO (2017) has emphasised that accessible and affordable rehabilitation plays a fundamental role in ensuring healthy lives and promoting well-being for all ages (Sustainable Development Goal). Health promotion can be considered on three levels –primary, secondary and tertiary prevention:

● Primary prevention seeks to prevent the onset of disease through healthy living. It is achieved by health education and lifestyle and behavioural changes.

- Secondary prevention aims to stop or slow disease progression and prevent complications through early diagnosis and adequate treatment.
- Tertiary prevention is focused on reducing impairments and activity restrictions.

All health professionals have a role to play in enabling people to return to meaningful roles in the wider community with a focus on health and wellness, rather than a focus mainly on ill health and disability (Cott et al 2007; Dean 2009). Ultimately this means that rehabilitation involves changing behaviour.

Diseases like hypertension and diabetes mellitus may be prevented (first-degree prevention) or, if present, may be controlled (second-degree prevention) through regular exercise, thus preventing other diseases (stroke or heart attack). Therapists are well equipped to promote health and participation across all levels of prevention through identifying, modifying and encouraging appropriate enjoyable exercises and physical activities for patients.

CONCLUSIONS

Therapists have a key role to play in enabling patients to experience and relearn optimal movement and function in everyday life within the constraints imposed by neurological disease and presenting impairments. This chapter has discussed 10 principles to guide current clinical practice in neurorehabilitation: the ICF, team work, patient-centred care, prediction, neural plasticity, a systems model of motor control, functional movement re-education, skill acquisition, self-management (self-efficacy) and health promotion. As well as focusing on the physical activities required to re-educate movement and promote skill acquisition, therapists need to understand how to facilitate behavioural change by promoting self-efficacy and enhancing their patients' self-management skills. Components selected within therapy sessions should be evidence based rather than based on therapist preference for a specific treatment approach. More research is required to understand which patient responds best to which interventions and to determine optimal dose, intensity and timing. It is crucial to link clinical practice to quality research.

This chapter is an abridged version adapted from Lennon and Bassile (2018) with permission.

References

Ackerley, S.J., Stinear, C.M., Barber, P.A., Byblow, W.D., 2014. Priming sensorimotor cortex to enhance task-specific training after subcortical stroke. Clinical Neurophysiology 125, 1451–1458.

Bandura, A., 1997. The nature and structure of self-efficacy. In: Bandura A Self-efficacy: the exercise of control. W.H Freeman and Company, New York.

Barron, C.J., Klaber Moffett, J.A., Potter, M. 2007. Patient expectations of physiotherapy: definitions, concepts and theories. Physiotherapy Theory and Practice 23, 37–46.

Birkenmeier, R.L., Prager, E.M., Lang, C.E., 2010. Translating animal doses of task-specific training to people with chronic stroke in one hour therapy sessions: a proof of concept study. Neurorehabilitation Neural Repair 24 (7), 620–635.

Brazzelli, M., Saunders, D.H., et al., 2012. Physical fitness training for patients with stroke: updated review. Stroke 43, e39–e40. https://doi.org/10.1161/STROKEAHA.111.647008.

Bright, F.A.S., Kayes, N.M., McCann, C.M., McPherson, K.M., 2011. Understanding hope after stroke: a systematic review of the literature using concept analysis. Topics in Stroke Rehabilitation 18 (5), 490–508.

Bovend'Eerdt, T.J.H., Botell, R.E., Wade, D.T., 2009. Writing SMART rehabilitation goals and achieving goal attainment scaling: a practical guide. Clinical Rehabilitation 23, 352–361.

Braun, S.M., Beurskens, A.J., Borm, P.J., et al., 2006. The effects of mental practice in stroke rehabilitation. Archives of Physical Medicine and Rehabilitation 87, 842–852.

Byblow, W.D., Stinear, C.M., Smith, M.C., et al., 2012. Mirror symmetric bimanual movement priming can increase corticomotor excitability and enhance motor learning. PLoS ONE 7 (3), e33882.

Carr, J.H., Shepherd, R.B., 2003. Stroke rehabilitation: guidelines for exercise and training to optimise motor skills. Butterworth Heinemann, Oxford.

Carr, J.H., Shepherd, J.H., 2006. Neurological rehabilitation. Disability & Rehabilitation 28, 811–812.

Cott, C.A., Wiles, R., Devitt, R., 2007. Continuity, transition and participation: preparing clients for life in the community post-stroke. Disability & Rehabilitation 29, 1566–1574.

Clarke, D.I., Forster, A., 2015. Improving post recovery: the role of the multi-disciplinary health care team. Journal of Multidisciplinary Health Care 8, 433–442.

Dayan, E., Cohen, L.G., 2011. Neuroplasticity subserving motor skill learning. Neuron 72, 443–454.

Dean, E., 2009. Foreword from the special issue editor of 'Physical Therapy Practice in the 21st Century: a new evidence-informed paradigm and implications. Physiotherapy Theory and Practice 25, 328–329.

Dean, C.M., Shepherd, R.B., 1997. Task-related training improves performance of seated reaching tasks after stroke. A randomized controlled trial. Stroke 28, 722–728.

Dean, C.M., Richards, C.L., Malouin, F., 2000. Task-related circuit training improves performance of locomotor tasks in chronic stroke: a randomized, controlled pilot trial. Archives Physical Medicine & Rehabilitation 81 (4), 409–417.

Dimyan, M.A., Cohen, L., 2011. Neuroplasticity in the context of motor rehabilitation after stroke. Nat Rev Neurology 7 (2), 76–85.

Dobkin, B.H., Firestine, A., et al., 2004. Ankle dorsiflexion as an fMRI paradigm to assay motor control for walking during rehabilitation. NeuroImage 23 (1), 370–381.

Fryer, C.E., et al., 2016. Self-management programmes for quality of life in people with stroke. Cochrane Database of Systematic Reviews (Issue 8) Art No; CD010442.

Fuller, C.R., 2016. Echoes of a closed door: a life lived following a stroke. Self-published. Available at: www.carolrfuller.com.

Garner, J., Lennon, S. 2018. Neurological assessment: the basis of clinical decision making (chapter 4). In: Lennon, S., Ramdharry, G., Verheyden, G. (Eds.), The Neurological Physiotherapy Pocketbook. second ed. Elsevier Science, London.

Gentile, A.M., 2000. Skill acquisition: action, movement and neuromotor processes. In: Carr, J., Shepherd, R. (Eds.), Movement science foundations for physical therapy in rehabilitation, second ed. Aspen Publishers, Maryland.

Health Foundation, 2014. Person-centred care made simple. Available at: http://person centredcare.health.org.uk.

Hordacre, B., McCambridge, A., 2018. Motor Control: Structure and Function of the Nervous System (chapter 2). In: Lennon, S., Ramdharry, G., Verheyden, G. (Eds.), The Neurological Physiotherapy Pocketbook, second ed. Elsevier Science, London.

Hornby, T.G., Straube, D.S., et al., 2011. Importance of specificity, amount, and intensity of locomotor training to improve ambulatory function in patients poststroke. Topics in Stroke Rehabilitation 18, 293–307.

Hubbard, I.J., Neil, C., Carey, L.M., 2009. Task-specific training: evidence for and translation into clinical practice. Occupational Therapy International 16, 175–189.

Jackson, P.L., Lafleur, M.F., Richards, C., et al., 2001. Potential role of mental practice using motor imagery in neurologic rehabilitation. Archives of Physical Medicine and Rehabilitation 82, 1133–1141.

Jones, F., Kulnik, S.T., 2018. Self-management (chapter 17). In: Lennon, S., Ramdharry, G. (Eds.), Verheyden G Physical Management for Neurological Conditions, fourth ed. Elsevier Science, London.

Keus, S., Munneke, M., Graziano, M., Paltamaa, J., et al., 2014. European Physiotherapy Guidelines for Parkinson's Disease. KNGf/ParkinsonNet, The Netherlands.

Kimberley, T.J., Novak, I., Boyd, L., Fowler, E., 2017. Stepping up to rethink the future of rehabilitation: IV STEP considerations and inspirations. Pediatric Physical Therapy S76–S85.

Kollen, B.J., Lennon, S., Lyons, B., Wheatley-Smith, L., Scheper, M., Buurke, J., Halfens, J., Geurts, A., Kwakkel, G., 2009. The effectiveness of the Bobath Concept in stroke rehabilitation: what is the evidence? Stroke 40, e89–e97.

Krishnan, S., York, M.K., Bacchus, D., Heyn, P.C., 2017. Coping with caregiver burnout when caring for a person with neurodegenerative diseases: a guide for caregivers. Archives Physical Medicine and Rehabilitation 98 (4), 805–807.

Kwakkel, G., 2006. Impact of intensity of practice after stroke: issues for consideration. Disability and Rehabilitation 28, 823–830.

Kwakkel, G., Kollen, B., Lindeman, E., 2004. Understanding the pattern of functional recovery after stroke. Restorative Neurology & Neuroscience 22, 281–299.

Laguna, P.L., 2000. The effect of model observation versus physical practice during motor skill acquisition and performance. Journal of Human Movement Studies 39, 171–191.

Lang, C.E., Lohse, K.E., Birkenmeier, R.E., 2015. Dose and timing in neurorehabilitation: prescribing motor therapy after stroke. Current Opinion in Neurology 28 (6), 549–555.

Lennon, S., Bassile, C., 2018. Guiding principles of neurological (chapter 1). In: Lennon, S., Ramdharry, G., Verheyden, G. (Eds.), Physical Management for Neurological Conditions, fourth ed. Elsevier Science, London.

Lennon, S., McKenna, S., Jones, F., 2013. Self-management programmes for people post stroke: a systematic review. Clinical Rehabilitation 27 (10), 867–878.

Levin, M.F., Kleim, J.A., Wolf, S.L., 2009. What do motor recovery and compensation mean in patients following stroke? Neurorehabilitation and Neural Repair 23, 313–319.

McDonnell, M.N., Koblar, S., Ward, N.S., et al., 2015. An investigation of cortical neuroplasticity following stroke in adults: is there evidence for a critical window for rehabilitation? BMC Neurology 15, 109.

Muratori, L.M., Lamberg, E.M., Quinn, L., Duff, S.V., 2013. Applying principles of motor learning and control to upper extremity rehabilitation. Journal of Hand Therapy 26 (2), 94–103.

NHS England, 2016. Realising the value. Ten key actions to put people and communities at the heart of health and wellbeing. NHS England, London.

Nithianantharajah, J., Hannan, A.J., 2006. Enriched environments, experience-dependent plasticity and disorders of the nervous system. Nature Reviews Neuroscience 7, 697–709.

Nilsen, D.M., Gillen, G., Gordon, A.M., 2010. Use of mental practice to improve upper limb recovery after stroke: a systematic review. American Journal of Occupational Therapy 64, 695–708.

Nudo, R.J., 2013. Recovery after brain injury: mechanisms and principles. Frontiers in Human Neuroscience 7, 887. https://doi.org/10.3389.

Peurala, S.H., Karttunen, A.H., et al., 2014. Evidence for the effectiveness of walking training on walking and self-care after stroke: a systematic review and meta-analysis of randomized controlled trials. Journal of Rehabilitation Medicine 46, 387–399.

Playford, E.D., Siegert, R., Levack, W., Freeman, J., 2009. Areas of consensus and controversy about goal setting in rehabilitation: a conference report. Clinical Rehabilitation 23, 334–344.

Pollock, A., Baer, G., Campbell, P., Choo, P.L., Forster, A., Morris, J., Pomeroy, V.M., Langhorne, P., 2014. Physical rehabilitation approaches for the recovery of function and mobility following stroke. Cochrane Database Systematic Reviews (4), CD001920.

Reo, J.A., Mercer, V.S., 2004. Effects of live, videotaped or written instruction on learning an upper-extremity exercise program. Physical Therapy 84 (7), 622–633.

Schmidt, R., Lee, T., 2013. Motor Learning and Performance, 5E With Web Study Guide: From Principles to Application. Human Kinetics, Illinois.

Shumway Cook, A., Woollacott, M.H., 2017. Motor control: translating research into clinical practice. 5th edition. Williams & Wilkins, Baltimore.

Sidaway, B., Ahn, S., Boldeau, P., Griffin, S., Noyes, B., Pelletier, K., 2008. A comparison of manual guidance and knowledge of results in the learning of a weight-bearing skill. Journal of Neurologic Physical Therapy 32 (1), 32.

Stroke Unit Trialists Collaboration (SUTC), 2013. Organised inpatient (stroke unit) care for stroke (review). Cochrane Database Systematic Reviews 9, CD000197.

Van Vliet, P., Wulf, G., 2006. Extrinsic feedback for motor learning after stroke: what is the evidence? Disability & Rehabilitation 28, 831–840.

Verbeek, J.M., Van Wegen, E.E.H., Van Peppen RRs, Hendriks, H.J.M., et al., 2014. KNGF Clinical Practice Guideline for Physical Therapy in patients with stroke. Royal Dutch Society for Physical Therapy, the Netherlands.

Wade, D.T., 2009. Goal setting in rehabilitation: an overview of what, why and how. Clin Rehabil. 23, 291–295.

Whalley Hammell, K., 2009. The wider context of neurorehabilitation. In: Lennon, S., Stokes, M. (Eds.), Pocketbook of Neurological Physiotherapy. Elsevier Science, London.

WHO, 2001. International Classification of Functioning, Disability and Health (ICF). World Health Organization, Geneva. Available online at: http://www.who.int/classifications/icf/en/. Last accessed on May 10, 2018.

WHO, 2017. Rehab 2030: a call for action. Available at: http://www.who.int/disabilities/care/rehab-2030/en/.

Williams, M., Hodges, N.J., 2004. Skill acquisition in sport: research, theory and practice. Routledge, London.

Winstein, C.J., 1991. Designing practice for motor learning: clinical implications. In: Lister, M.J. (Ed.), Contemporary management of motor control problems: proceedings of the II STEP Conference. Foundation for Physical Therapy, Alexandria, Virginia.

Winstein, C.J., Pohl, P.S., Lewthwaite, R., 1994. Effects of physical guidance and knowledge of results on motor learning: support for the guidance hypothesis. Research Quarterly for Exercise and Sport 64 (4), 316–323.

Winstein, C.J., Lewthwaite, R., Blanton, S.R., Wolf, L.B., Wishart, L., 2014. Infusing motor learning research into neurorehabilitation practice: a historical perspective with case exemplar from the accelerated skill acquisition program. Journal of Neurologic Physical Therapy 38, 190–200.

Wulf, G., 2013. Attentional focus and motor learning: a review of 15 years. International Journal of Sport and Exercise Psychology 6, 77–104.

Wulf, G., Lewthwaite, R., 2016. Optimizing performance through intrinsic motivation and attention for learning: The OPTIMAL theory of motor learning. Psychological Bulletin Rev 23, 1382–1414.

CHAPTER 2

Motor control: structure and function of the nervous system

Brenton Hordacre and Alana McCambridge

INTRODUCTION

Motor control is the process of activating, coordinating and regulating mechanisms essential for the production of functional movements. Abnormalities of motor control can become evident for various neurological presentations. Understanding human motor control may assist therapists in selecting appropriate clinical interventions and design of rehabilitation programs. This chapter outlines major theories of motor control whilst highlighting how the motor system is organised and important structures involved in upper and lower limb movement. As a quick reference for clinicians, the effect of lesion location within the motor system is provided. The concept of neuroplasticity is introduced as a mechanism to facilitate recovery of motor function following injury. Finally, a brief summary of how transcranial magnetic stimulation (TMS) can be used to probe the motor system is provided.

THEORIES OF MOTOR CONTROL

Several theories of motor control are outlined in Box 2.1. Each theory provides an interpretation of how movement is generated. These theories place differing levels of significance on various neural structures and mechanisms involved in motor control. For a summary of the limitations and clinical implications of each theory, refer to Shumway-Cook (2012).

STRUCTURE AND FUNCTION OF THE MOTOR SYSTEM

To understand how the human motor system produces voluntary movement, it is important to understand the organization of the nervous system (Fig. 2.1).

The central nervous system includes neural structures in the brain and spinal cord. The brain consists of the cerebrum, brainstem and cerebellum. The brainstem can be subdivided into the midbrain, pons and medulla. The cerebrum contains the cerebral cortex and subcortical structures such as the basal ganglia, thalamus and hippocampus. Each hemisphere of the cerebral cortex can be divided into the frontal, parietal, occipital and temporal lobes (shown in Fig. 2.2) and is

Box 2.1 Theories of motor control

- **Reflex Theory** – a series of reflex responses to a stimulus which combine to form the basis for functional movement.
- **Hierarchical Theories** – motor control is organised in a top-down structure with higher association areas exerting control over cortical regions followed by the spinal level.
- **Motor Programming Theories** – movement is produced by a central motor pattern.
- **Systems Theory** – movement is produced by the synergistic interaction of multiple systems which are influenced by both internal and external factors.
- **Dynamic Action Theories** – movement results from the interaction between components of the motor system without requiring specific commands or motor programs.
- **Ecological Theories** – detecting information in the environment relevant to movement will guide actions.

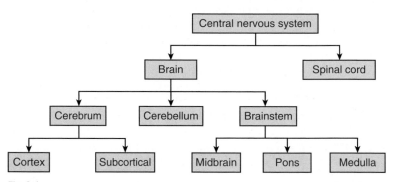

Fig. 2.1
Divisions of the central nervous system.

functionally organised into specialised areas such as the motor, somatosensory, visual, auditory, gustatory and olfactory cortices and associated areas. The motor cortex is primarily responsible for the execution of motor commands and is there-fore important for motor control. A summary of key features of the motor cortex is provided in Box 2.2. Cortical regions can also be classified by their cytoarchitecture, termed *Brodmann areas* (Box 2.3).

The peripheral nervous system consists of neurons located outside the central nervous system, such as afferent neurons (axon of a sensory neuron) that carry afferent signals *to the central nervous system* and efferent neurons (axon of a motor

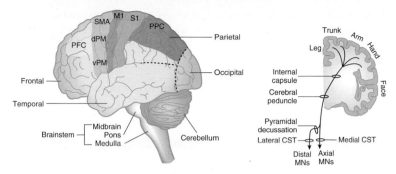

Fig. 2.2
(Left) Lateral view of the left hemisphere showing key cortical areas for voluntary movement. Each hemisphere contains the frontal, parietal, occipital and temporal lobe. Regions within these lobes are further separated based on functional specialisation. PFC, prefrontal cortex; dPM, Dorsal premotor area; M1, primary motor cortex; PPC, posterior parietal cortex; S1, primary sensory cortex; SMA, supplementary motor area; vPM, ventral premotor area. (Right) Coronal view showing the somatotopic organisation of M1 and schematic representation of the lateral and medial corticospinal tract (CST) projecting to distal and axial motor neurones (MNs).

Box 2.2 Important features of the primary motor cortex

- Motor cortical areas are somatotopically organised, essentially subdivided between the face, arm and leg but with broad overlapping areas (Rathelot & Strick 2006).
- The face and hand have disproportionately large representations because of the greatest need for precision and control of these areas (refer to Fig. 2.2, right).
- The motor cortex is thought to represent a map of movements (Georgopoulos et al 1982) or spatial locations to which movements are directed (Graziano et al 2002, Stefan et al 2004), rather than the control of individual muscles.

Box 2.3 Cortical areas important for motor control

Frontal lobe	
Primary motor cortex (M1)	Brodmann area 4
Supplementary motor cortex (SMA)	Brodmann area 6
Premotor area (PM)	Brodmann area 6, 8
Prefrontal cortex (PFC), dorsolateral	Brodmann area 9, 46
Parietal lobe	
Primary somatosensory cortex (S1)	Brodmann area 1, 2, 3
Posterior parietal cortex (PPC)	Brodmann area 5, 7

neurone) that carry signals *from the central nervous system.* Efferent neurons can be classified as somatic or autonomic. Somatic motor neurones control skeletal musculature and are under voluntary control, whereas autonomic motor neurones control internal organs, blood vessels and glands that are not under voluntary control.

VOLUNTARY MOVEMENT

Goal-directed voluntary movements can be achieved through three phases: planning, initiation and execution. The main areas involved in each phase are shown in Box 2.4.

Box 2.4 Motor system hierarchy

Planning	Prefrontal cortex and Posterior parietal cortex	Decision to move is created and converted into possible motor commands based on current body position and visual information.
Initiation	Premotor and supplementary motor areas	Motor commands are devised and maintained until needed.
	Basal ganglia	Motor commands are refined and unsuitable movements prevented.
Execution	Motor cortex and Spinal cord	Motor commands are released and transmitted via descending motor pathways.

Motor Control Hierarchy

Motor control research suggests there is a hierarchical level of processing in addition to parallel loops that process information simultaneously. Within the hierarchy, high levels of function control decision making and strategy (e.g. association areas, basal ganglia), whereas low levels are concerned with motor execution (e.g. brainstem, spinal cord). Hierarchical and parallel control ensures there is a level of redundancy in the system, which is important for multitasking and complex sequential movements and may be useful for recovery of function after neural injury.

An overview of the motor system is shown in Fig. 2.3. Motor commands from the cortex are transmitted through descending motor pathways directly or indirectly via the brainstem to alpha motor neurones and interneurons in the spinal cord (see Fig. 2.3, solid black lines). The lateral corticospinal tract is the principal motor pathway for transmitting descending motor commands to distal limb muscles. In the medulla 75% to 90% of axons in the lateral corticospinal tract decussate (Kuypers 1964, Rosenzweig et al 2009); therefore motor areas in the right hemisphere control the left side of the body and vice versa. Activated motor neurones in the spinal cord carry neural signals to the skeletal musculature, causing the muscles to contract and produce movement.

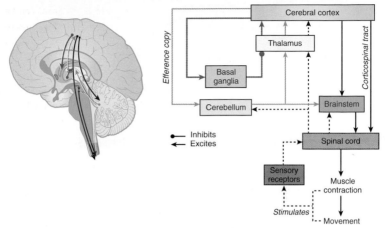

Fig. 2.3
Schematic overview of the motor system, showing the cortico-basal-ganglia-thalamo-cortical loop (dark gray line) and cortico-cerebello-thalamo-cortical loop (light gray line). Medial view of the right hemisphere shown, including cerebellum, brainstem and spinal cord. Arrows indicate excitatory influence; circles indicate inhibitory influence. Dashed lines indicate afferent input.

Sensory Feedback

Movement is detected by sensory receptors located in the muscles and joints. Proprioceptive feedback is also processed hierarchically and integrated with other sensory sources. At the lowest level, sensory feedback forms spinal reflex loops. At higher levels, sensory feedback may be integrated in the somatosensory cortex via the thalamus and transmitted to the cerebellum, where it is compared with motor output from the cortex (see Fig. 2.3, dashed lines).

Role of the Cerebellum

A copy of the descending motor command is transmitted from the cortex to the cerebellum, termed the *efference copy* (see Fig. 2.3, light gray line). The cerebellum compares the efference copy to the sensory input (i.e. intended movement versus actual movement), returns this information to the cortex and, if necessary, adjusts the motor output to reduce movement errors. This parallel level of processing is called the **cortico-cerebello-thalamo-cortical** loop (see Fig. 2.3, light gray lines) and is particularly important during motor learning, as untrained movements produce many errors that are corrected through practice.

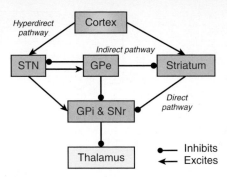

Fig. 2.4
Schematic of the hyperdirect, indirect and direct pathway of the basal ganglia. GPe, Globus pallidus externus; GPi, globus pallidus internus; SNr, substantia nigra; STN, subthalamic nucleus. Adapted from Nambu et al (2002).

Role of the Basal Ganglia

The basal ganglia are a group of interconnected subcortical nuclei consisting of the striatum (caudate nucleus + putamen), globus pallidus (internal + external segments), substantia nigra and subthalamic nucleus. The basal ganglia shape and select motor output through the **cortico-basal-ganglia-thalamo-cortical loop** (see Fig. 2.3, dark gray lines). The striatum is the major input nucleus to the basal ganglia, receiving excitatory inputs from the motor cortex, supplementary motor area and premotor areas. The striatum projects to the internal globus pallidus directly or indirectly via the external globus pallidus and substantia nigra, respectively, forming the direct and indirect pathways (Fig. 2.4, adapted from Nambu et al 2002). The main output nuclei of the basal ganglia are the internal globus pallidus and substantia nigra, which tonically inhibit the thalamus. Activation of the direct pathway disinhibits the thalamus, thereby increasing thalamocortical drive. In contrast, the indirect pathway further inhibits the thalamus and decreases thalamocortical drive. The hyperdirect pathway is thought to widely inhibit the thalamus, and delayed activity via the direct and indirect pathway acts to release only the desired motor output (Nambu et al 2002). As a result, the direct pathway facilitates movement or desired motor plans, whereas the indirect pathway inhibits movement or competing motor plans.

UPPER LIMB MOVEMENT

There are several important features specific to neural control of the upper limb. For example, reaching and grasping are mediated through separate but parallel routes from the visual cortex. Visual information about the location of the target is needed for reaching, whereas information about the shape is needed for

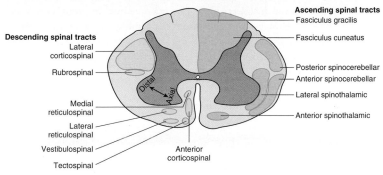

Fig. 2.5
Ascending (sensory) and descending (motor) tracts shown on separate sides of the spinal cord in the transverse plane. Axial and distal motor nuclei are arranged medial to lateral in the ventral horn of the spinal cord.

grasping. The motor cortex primarily processes aspects of reaching in the dorsal premotor area and for grasping in the ventral premotor area. Within the ventral premotor area, individual neurons may specifically encode a type of task, such as precision grip or power grip (Rizzolatti et al 1996). Evolutionary changes in the corticospinal tract, such as direct monosynaptic connections and increased number of corticospinal neurons, are thought to underlie the ability of humans to perform individual finger movements (Lemon 2008).

Axial and distal muscles are preferentially controlled through medial and lateral motor pathways, respectively. In the spinal cord, motor neurones are arranged along a medial-to-lateral axis, whereby axial muscles are located in the ventromedial portion, distal limb muscles are located in the dorsolateral portion and proximal limb muscles in between (Fig. 2.5). Medial motor pathways terminate bilaterally in the left and right ventromedial horns of the spinal cord. Lateral motor pathways terminate in the dorsolateral horn on the contralateral side. Therefore axial and proximal muscles are controlled bilaterally by contralateral and ipsilateral motor areas, whereas distal limb muscles are primarily controlled by contralateral motor areas. However, there is evidence to suggest that ipsilateral motor areas do contribute to distal upper limb movements of more complex motor tasks (Chen et al 1997).

Bimanual and unimanual movements require interhemispheric communication via the corpus callosum. To perform a unimanual or asymmetrical bimanual task, the contralateral motor cortex inhibits activity of the opposite motor cortex to prevent unwanted mirror movements and permit each limb to move independently (Carson 2005). Rhythmic bimanual movements in an asymmetrical pattern can be successfully achieved at slower speeds (for example, rubbing your tummy and patting your head). However, at faster speeds the stability of the motor system is perturbed and spontaneous transitions to mirror symmetrical movement patterns are frequently observed (Haken et al 1985). Key features of upper limb movement are summarised in Box 2.5.

Box 2.5 Key features for upper limb movement

- Reaching and grasping requires precise spatiotemporal control of proximal and distal upper limb muscles to perform a smooth and coordinated movement.
- Visual information encoding the location and shape of an object is important for motor planning.
- Axial muscles receive bilateral inputs from both motor cortices, whereas distal muscles primarily receive direct corticospinal input from the contralateral motor cortex.
- Between-hemisphere communication via the corpus callosum allows each arm to move independent of the other.

LOWER LIMB MOVEMENT

The trunk and lower limbs play a vital role in static balance, dynamic balance and locomotion. The trunk is considered the central point of the body, with proximal trunk control required for lower limb movements to keep the body in an upright position and adjust weight shift to keep or return the centre of mass within the base of support to prevent falling (Davies 1990). Given its relative mass and height, the trunk acts as an inverted pendulum, with positional adjustments vital to help maintain balance and counter postural disturbances. The control of body position is achieved through an interplay of feedforward and feedback reflexes, which respectively anticipate or respond, to postural disturbance (Fig. 2.6). Impairments in trunk control have been shown to affect both balance and gait after stroke (Karatas et al 2004, Verheyden et al 2006), suggesting the trunk could be a potential therapeutic target for rehabilitation.

Motor control of the lower limbs and trunk are important for locomotion, which is a basic human function and provides the capability to move the centre of gravity in a desired direction. Locomotion is achieved through a coordinated, rhythmic and alternating step pattern which progresses the centre of gravity forward within the base of support provided by the lower limbs.

Several components of the central nervous system contribute to motor control of the lower limbs. These can be separated into spinal and supraspinal components.

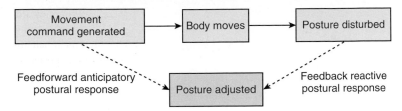

Fig. 2.6
Feedforward and feedback postural responses.

Contribution from the spinal cord was identified over 100 years ago, where it was reported that cats with spinal lesions were able to achieve normal locomotion patterns (Brown 1911). Commands can be generated sequentially in time during each step by neural networks located in the spinal cord called *central pattern generators* (Grillner et al 1991, Lacquaniti et al 2012). Central pattern generators behave like motor programs and have the capacity to generate complex, but stereotypical, patterns of motor output in the absence of supraspinal or sensory input (Grillner & Wallen 1985, Jordan 1998). Reaction to pertubations introduced during gait, such as stumbling on an obstacle, can be rapidly responded to through spinal reflexes (Dietz 1987) (Fig. 2.7).

Several additional systems are known to influence spinal central pattern generators and provide descending control of lower limb movement (Jahn et al 2008). Descending pathways from higher centres integrate sensory feedback from the periphery and allow variation and adaptability in locomotor patterns to meet environment and task demands (Jordan 1998, Nielsen 2003). The cortex, brainstem and cerebellum provide input via the lateral corticospinal tract and lateral reticulospinal tract to modify and adapt the gait patterns for the required task (Duysens & Van de Crommert 1998). Several studies highlight the importance of the cortex for lower limb motor control in humans, which potentially reflects more complex bipedal gait patterns (Fukuyama et al 1997, Porter & Lemon 1993). It is thought that the motor cortex has a role in timing of muscle activity during gait (Capaday et al 1999). The brainstem is thought to regulate speed and pacemakers for gait initiation (Jahn et al 2008). The cerebellar contribution to gait can be distinguished by the three anatomical regions of the cerebellum. The vermis regulates dynamic balance and rhythmic flexor/extensor activity; the spinocerebellum controls timing, amplitude and trajectory of movement; and the pontocerebellum is responsible for adjusting the locomotor pattern during complex situations (Ilg et al 2008, Morton & Bastian 2007). Key regions involved in motor control of the lower limb are shown in Fig. 2.7 and a summary is provided in Box 2.6.

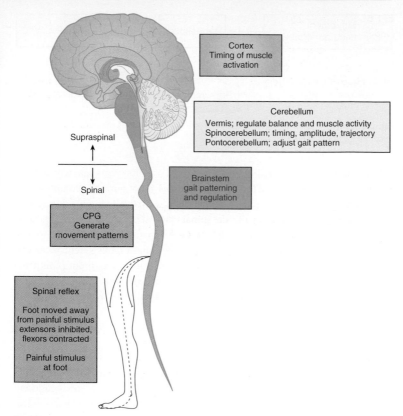

Fig. 2.7
Spinal and supraspinal contributions to lower limb motor control and production of gait. CPG, *Central pattern generator.*

Box 2.6 Key features for lower limb movement

- Trunk control is a key feature of lower limb movement, acting as a stable platform and adjusting the centre of gravity to maintain balance.
- Central pattern generators in the spinal cord behave like motor programs and have capacity to generate rhythmic, stereotypical movement of the lower limbs.
- Supraspinal structures provide descending input to modify and adapt the gait patterns for the required task.

EFFECT OF LESION LOCATION

Understanding which structures in the central nervous system contribute to the production of voluntary movement is important for identifying potential impairments when a lesion or dysfunction occurs to that region of the brain or spinal cord. Knowledge of the lesion location and therefore the expected impairments may assist therapists in designing appropriate rehabilitation programs to help restore function. Table 2.1 provides a basic summary of various structures that contribute to motor control and symptoms that may be evident after a lesion in these regions.

Table 2.1 Motor control in the central nervous system

Structure and function	Features/roles in movement generation	Effects of lesions
Cerebral cortex ● Initiation and modulation of movement	● Primary motor cortex: Executes voluntary movements ● Supplementary motor area: Movement initiation and planning of bimanual tasks and sequential movement, orientation of head and eyes. Important for learning new tasks. ● Premotor cortex: Movement planning and preparation. Controls trunk and girdle muscles. ● Primary somatosensory cortex: Receives sensory input. Identifies target location relative to body position. Discrimination of size/shape/texture. ● Posterior parietal cortex: Links motivation, interest and action. Integrates multimodal sensory information. ● Prefrontal cortex: Goal planning and strategy selection	● Contralateral paralysis or weakness (primary motor cortex) ● Apraxia, inability to initiate movement. Problem using internal cues (supplementary motor area) ● Mild paresis, slow, complex movements. Problem using external cues (premotor cortex) ● Decreased or loss of sensation (primary somatosensory cortex) ● Inability to discriminate tactile stimuli (primary somatosensory cortex) ● Problems with body image and visuospatial perception e.g. neglect (posterior parietal cortex) ● Problems with planning, attention and problem solving (prefrontal cortex)

Continued

2

Table 2.1 Motor control in the central nervous system—cont'd

Structure and function	Features/roles in movement generation	Effects of lesions
Basal ganglia ● Selects voluntary movement ● Movement sequencing ● Terminates movement	● Direct pathway: Excitatory, enables movement ● Indirect pathway: Inhibitory, slows or stops movement ● Interaction of direct and indirect pathway refines motor commands	● Akinesia/hypokinesia ● Bradykinesia ● Chorea ● Resting tremor ● Dystonia ● Rigidity ● Tics
Cerebellum ● Coordinates movement and postural control ● Regulates and adjusts movement to match intended motor plan	● Influences movement via motor areas of the cortex or the brainstem ● Balance and eye movement regulated by the vestibulocerebellum ● Gross limb movement regulated by the spinocerebellum ● Distal limb movement regulated by the cerebrocerebellum	● Unilateral lesions affect ipsilesional side of body ● Ataxia (common to all lesions of cerebellum) **Lesion of vestibulocerebellum** ● Nystagmus, disequilibrium, difficulty maintaining balance **Lesion of spinocerebellum** ● Limb ataxia, including dysdiadochokinesia, dysmetria, action tremor ● Gait ataxia **Lesion of cerebrocerebellum** ● Intention tremor ● Dysarthria
Brainstem ● Pyramidal tracts descend through brainstem ● Extrapyramidal tracts originate in brainstem ● Motor and sensory innervation to face and neck (cranial nerves)	**Corticospinal pathways (pyramidal tracts)** ● Corticospinal tract: Passes through but not modified by brainstem. Axons decussate in the medulla. ● Corticobulbar tract: Synapse with cranial nerve nuclei in brainstem and innervate muscles of head and neck ● Corticopontine tract: Synapse with nuclei in pons ● Corticoreticular tract: Synapse within reticular formation	● Abnormalities of cranial nerve function (speech, swallowing, visual disturbance, sensation of face and neck) ● Tone and postural abnormalities ● Upper motor neurone (UMN) syndrome ● Loss of visual tracking ● Increased extensor tone ● Impaired anticipatory postural adjustments

Table 2.1 Motor control in the central nervous system—cont'd

Structure and function	Features/roles in movement generation	Effects of lesions
	Brainstem pathways (extrapyramidal tracts) ● Vestibulospinal tract: Balance and postural control ● Reticulospinal tract: Medial tract facilitates movement and increases tone. Lateral tract inhibits movement and reduces tone. ● Rubrospinal tract: Fine hand movement ● Tectospinal tract: Head movement in relation to visual stimuli	
Spinal cord ● Spinal reflexes ● Central pattern generators ● Ascending and descending tracts	**Descending tracts (motor)** ● Lateral tracts: Lateral corticospinal tract, rubrospinal tract ● Medial tracts: Reticulospinal tract, vestibulospinal tract, anterior corticospinal tract **Ascending tracts (sensory)** ● Dorsal column/medial lemniscus system: Fasciculus gracilis, fasciculus cuneatus ● Anterolateral system: Lateral and anterior spinothalamic tract ● Spinocerebellar tracts: Anterior and posterior	● Sensory loss ● Upper motor neurone syndrome: paresis, spasticity e.g. exaggerated stretch reflexes, clonus

(Extracted from Shumway-Cook 2012 and Lundy-Ekman 2009).

NEUROPLASTICITY

In neurological rehabilitation, the purpose of therapy is often to improve function and control of movement. Relatively permanent changes in motor control and behaviour require practice and learning (Schmidt & Lee 2013) and are underpinned by the physiological process of neuroplasticity. Neuroplasticity is defined as the ability of the nervous system to respond to intrinsic and extrinsic stimuli by reorganisation of structure or function. It can occur on many levels, including molecular, cellular and across broad networks. The process of neuroplasticity occurs throughout life, but is facilitated during critical periods, including early development, periods of learning (Adkins et al 2006), environmental challenges and in response to disease or injury (Nudo 2013). Several studies have demonstrated that neuroplasticity plays a significant role in functional recovery and amelioration of impairment for a wide spectrum of brain diseases and injury (Grefkes & Fink 2011, Koski et al 2004, Nudo 2013).

Several indirect approaches are available to quantify neuroplasticity in humans. These include neuroimaging (e.g. functional magnetic resonance imaging, electroencephalography), noninvasive brain stimulation (transcranial magnetic stimulation [TMS]; described later) and behavioural outcome measures. From a clinical perspective, monitoring functional recovery with behavioural outcome measures may allow for identification of adaptive neuroplasticity responses. However, not all neuroplasticity responses are considered beneficial, and in some instances may in fact be detrimental to recovery (Madhavan et al 2010). Where improvements in behaviour are observed, the neuroplastic response is considered to be adaptive (Cohen et al 1997). Adaptive neuroplasticity is distinct from compensatory behaviours which describe alternative strategies to perform a particular movement or response (Levin et al 2008). Several characteristics are associated with adaptive neuroplasticity in rehabilitation (Box 2.7), and where possible, therapists should attempt to facilitate an environment that fosters neuroplasticity.

Box 2.7 Principles of neuroplasticity for clinicians

- Neuroplasticity is use dependent and specific
  - Nonuse or decreased sensory input may degrade function and decrease the size of cortical representations (Merzenich et al 1984, Werhahn et al 2002)
  - Neuroplasticity occurs within specific networks activated by therapy (Adkins et al 2006, Nudo et al 1996)
  - Task-specific rehabilitation can induce greater functional gains (Winstein et al 2004)
- Repetition and intensity influence neuroplasticity
  - Repetition is required for lasting neural changes (Kleim et al 2004, Monfils & Teskey 2004)
  - Greater intensity shown to induce neuroplasticity (Kleim et al 2002, Luke et al 2004)
- Neuroplasticity is time sensitive
  - Neuroplasticity occurs in different forms across training (Adkins et al 2006)
  - Neuroplasticity may be more amenable early after injury (McDonnell et al 2015)

Box 2.7 Principles of neuroplasticity for clinicians—cont'd

- Neuroplasticity is influenced by salience, motivation, feedback and attention
  - Greater neuroplastic response when training relevant and important tasks (Plautz et al 2000, Remple et al 2001)
  - Appropriate feedback can increase therapy quality and facilitate adaptive neuroplasticity (Van Vliet & Wulf 2006)
  - Attention and focus during training influence the capacity to learn (Wulf 2013)
- Strongly influenced by features of the environment
  - Enhanced sensory, cognitive, motor and social stimulation facilitate increased neuroplasticity and learning (Nithianantharajah & Hannan 2006)
- Neuroplasticity is influenced by adjuvant or adjunct therapies
  - Therapies which 'prime' the motor system facilitate greater neuroplastic response (Ackerley et al 2014, Byblow et al 2012)
  - Priming therapies include motor imagery, mental practice, sensory priming, movement-based priming, stimulation-based therapy or pharmacology (Stoykov & Madhavan 2015)
- Neuroplasticity is influenced by patient characteristics
  - Younger people exhibit a greater and more efficient neuroplastic response compared with older people (Markus et al 2005, Todd et al 2010)
  - Genetic profiles influence neuroplastic response (Antal et al 2010, Cheeran et al 2008)
  - Stress can impair neuroplasticity (Hordacre et al 2016, Sale et al 2008)
- Pharmacology influences neuroplasticity
  - GABA receptor agonists (e.g. baclofen, benzodiazepine; used for anxiety, seizures, spasticity) reduce neuroplasticity (Willerslev-Olsen et al 2011, Ziemann et al 2001)

WHAT CAN WE LEARN FROM TRANSCRANIAL MAGNETIC STIMULATION?

TMS is a noninvasive brain stimulation tool that can be used to artificially excite motor pathways and neural circuits in the human brain. TMS is commonly used in stroke research to investigate neurophysiological changes throughout recovery and in response to therapy interventions. There exists a wide range of stimulation protocols capable of examining many important aspects of motor function, such as corticomotor excitability, intracortical inhibition and sensorimotor integration, to name a few (Table 2.2, refer to Wassermann et al 2008 for more details).

After a stroke, stimulation over the ipsilesional motor cortex can determine the functional integrity of the corticospinal tract. If a single TMS pulse can produce a response (termed motor evoked potential) in the paretic limb, this indicates the ipsilesional corticospinal tract is at least partially intact and functionally capable of transmitting descending motor commands. A sequential algorithm has been developed as a prognostic tool to predict a patient's motor recovery potential

Table 2.2 Common TMS protocols applied to the motor system

What common TMS protocols can infer about the motor system		
Single-pulse TMS	Corticomotor excitability	Net excitability of intracortical interneurons, pyramidal neurons of the corticospinal tract and motor neurones in the spinal cord leading to the target muscle
	Cortical silent period	$GABA_B$–mediated inhibition in the cortex
	Motor mapping	Cortical representation of muscles
	Surround inhibition	Motor overflow/selectivity of motor commands
Paired-pulse TMS	Intracortical inhibition	$GABA_A$–mediated inhibition in the cortex
	Intracortical facilitation	Glutamatergic facilitation in the cortex
Nerve-conditioned TMS	Afferent inhibition	Sensorimotor integration: Inhibition exerted from sensory cortex to motor cortex
	Paired-associative stimulation	Spike-timing–dependent synaptic plasticity
Dual-coil TMS	Interhemispheric inhibition/facilitation	Inhibition exerted via the corpus callosum to the opposite motor cortex
	Cerebellar brain inhibition	Inhibition exerted from the cerebellum to motor cortex
	Premotor inhibition/ facilitation	Inhibition exerted from the ipsilateral or contralateral premotor area to the motor cortex
Repetitive TMS	Artificial lesioning	Temporary 'lesion' of an area to determine its involvement in a task
	Neuromodulation	Transiently increase or decrease excitability of target area

TMS, Transcranial magnetic stimulation.

(Stinear et al 2012). The algorithm uses single-pulse TMS to determine the presence or absence of motor evoked potentials in conjunction with clinical measures of function and neural imaging if necessary. Greater insight into the recovery potential of a given patient can help therapists deliver more targeted rehabilitation and set appropriate rehabilitation goals (Stinear et al 2017).

Another potential clinical application of TMS is as a neuromodulatory tool. Repetitive TMS delivers several hundred pulses at a low (1–4 Hz) or high (5–20 Hz) frequency to transiently increase or decrease corticospinal excitability, respectively (Wassermann et al 2008). Because the effects of repetitive TMS on corticospinal excitability outlast the period of stimulation, there is evidence to suggest these changes resemble synaptic plasticity and can enhance motor learning (Wassermann et al 2008), though early clinical trials are yet to support this (Hao et al 2013). To date, more evidence is needed to determine the efficacy of repetitive TMS to prime the brain for therapy and augment stroke rehabilitation. Further investigation of the mechanisms and effects of these protocols is needed before they can be applied to clinical practice.

IMPLICATIONS FOR NEUROPHYSIOTHEARPY

Therapists should aim to optimise movement patterns and facilitate restitution of function after neurological injury. Understanding how the motor system controls particular aspects of normal and abnormal movement can provide the rationale for selecting appropriate rehabilitation strategies. Therefore components of the motor system must be considered in light of the neurological injury when designing therapy programs. Furthermore, rehabilitation is likely to be most effective when principles of neuroplasticity are considered (see Box 2.7), and, where possible, consideration should be given to tailor therapy and the environment to optimise the potential for functional improvements.

References

Ackerley, S.J., Stinear, C.M., Barber, P.A., Byblow, W.D., 2014. Priming sensorimotor cortex to enhance task-specific training after subcortical stroke. Clinical Neurophysiology 125, 1451–1458.

Adkins, D.L., Boychuk, J., Remple, M.S., Kleim, J.A., 2006. Motor training induces experience-specific patterns of plasticity across motor cortex and spinal cord. Journal of Applied Physiology 101, 1776–1782.

Antal, A., Chaieb, L., Moliadze, V., et al., 2010. Brain-derived neurotrophic factor (BDNF) gene polymorphisms shape cortical plasticity in humans. Brain Stimulation. 3, 230–237.

Brown, T.G., 1911. The intrinsic factors in the act of progression in the mammal. Proceedings of the Royal Society of London. Series B: Biological Sciences 84, 308–319.

Byblow, W.D., Stinear, C.M., Smith, M.C., et al., 2012. Mirror symmetric bimanual movement priming can increase corticomotor excitability and enhance motor learning. PLoS ONE 7(3): e33882.

Capaday, C., Lavoie, B.A., Barbeau, H., Schneider, C., Bonnard, M., 1999. Studies on the corticospinal control of human walking. I. Responses to focal transcranial magnetic stimulation of the motor cortex. Journal of Neurophysiology 81, 129–139.

Carson, R.G., 2005. Neural pathways mediating bilateral interactions between the upper limbs. Brain Research. Brain Research Reviews 49, 641–662.

Cheeran, B., Talelli, P., Mori, F., et al., 2008. A common polymorphism in the brain-derived neurotrophic factor gene (BDNF) modulates human cortical plasticity and the response to rTMS. Journal of Physiology 586, 5717–5725.

Chen, R., Gerloff, C., Hallett, M., Cohen, L.G., 1997. Involvement of the ipsilateral motor cortex in finger movements of different complexities. Annals of Neurology 41, 247–254.

Cohen, L.G., Celnik, P., Pascual-Leone, A., et al., 1997. Functional relevance of cross-modal plasticity in blind humans. Nature. 389, 180–183.

Davies, P.M., 1990. Problems associated with the loss of selective trunk activity in hemiplegia. In: Right in the middle: Selective trunk activity in the treatment of adult hemiplegia. Berlin, Heidelberg, Springer Berlin Heidelberg. p 31–65.

Dietz, V., 1987. Role of peripheral afferents and spinal reflexes in normal and impaired human locomotion. Revue Neurologique. (Paris) 143, 241–254.

Duysens, J., Van de Crommert, H.W., 1998. Neural control of locomotion; Part 1: the central pattern generator from cats to humans. Gait and Posture 7, 131–141.

Fukuyama, H., Ouchi, Y., Matsuzaki, S., et al., 1997. Brain functional activity during gait in normal subjects: a SPECT study. Neuroscience Letters 228, 183–186.

Georgopoulos, A.P., Kalaska, J.F., Caminiti, R., Massey, J.T., 1982. On the relations between the direction of two-dimensional arm movements and cell discharge in primate motor cortex. Journal of Neuroscience 2, 1527–1537.

Graziano, M.S., Taylor, C.S., Moore, T., 2002. Complex movements evoked by micro-stimulation of precentral cortex. Neuron. 34, 841–851.

Grefkes, C., Fink, G.R., 2011. Reorganization of cerebral networks after stroke: new insights from neuroimaging with connectivity approaches. Brain. 134, 1264–1276.

Grillner, S., Wallen, P., 1985. Central pattern generators for locomotion, with special reference to vertebrates. Annual Review of Neuroscience 8, 233–261.

Grillner, S., Wallen, P., Brodin, L., Lansner, A., 1991. Neuronal network generating locomotor behavior in lamprey: circuitry, transmitters, membrane properties, and simulation. Annual Review of Neuroscience 14, 169–199.

Haken, H., Kelso, J.A., Bunz, H., 1985. A theoretical model of phase transitions in human hand movements. Biological Cybernetics 51, 347–356.

Hao, Z., Wang, D., Zeng, Y., Liu, M., 2013. Repetitive transcranial magnetic stimulation for improving function after stroke. Cochrane Database of Systematic Reviews. 5, D008862.

Hordacre, B., Immink, M.A., Ridding, M.C., Hillier, S., 2016. Perceptual-motor learning benefits from increased stress and anxiety. Human Movement Science. 49, 36–46.

Ilg, W., Giese, M.A., Gizewski, E.R., Schoch, B., Timmann, D., 2008. The influence of focal cerebellar lesions on the control and adaptation of gait. Brain. 131, 2913–2927.

Jahn, K., Deutschländer, A., Stephan, T., et al., 2008. Imaging human supraspinal locomotor centers in brainstem and cerebellum. Neuroimage. 39, 786–792.

Jordan, L.M., 1998. Initiation of locomotion in mammals. Annals of the New York Academy of Sciences 860, 83–93.

Karatas, M., Cetin, N., Bayramoglu, M., Dilek, A., 2004. Trunk muscle strength in relation to balance and functional disability in unihemispheric stroke patients. American Journal of Physical Medicine & Rehabilitation 83, 81–87.

Kleim, J.A., Barbay, S., Cooper, N.R., et al., 2002. Motor learning-dependent synaptogenesis is localized to functionally reorganized motor cortex. Neurobiology of Learning and Memory 77, 63–77.

Kleim, J.A., Hogg, T.M., Vandenberg, P.M., et al., 2004. Cortical synaptogenesis and motor map reorganization occur during late, but not early, phase of motor skill learning. Journal of Neuroscience 24, 628–633.

Koski, L., Mernar, T.J., Dobkin, B.H., 2004. Immediate and long-term changes in corticomotor output in response to rehabilitation: correlation with functional improvements in chronic stroke. Neurorehabilitation and Neural Repair. 18, 230–249.

Kuypers, H.G., 1964. The descending pathways to the spinal cord, their anatomy and function. Progress in Brain Research 11, 178–202.

Lacquaniti, F., Ivanenko, Y.P., Zago, M., 2012. Development of human locomotion. Current Opinion in Neurobiology 22, 822–828.

Lemon, R.N., 2008. Descending pathways in motor control. Annual Review of Neuroscience 31, 195–218.

Levin, M.F., Kleim, J.A., Wolf, S.L., 2008. What do motor "recovery" and "compensation" mean in patients following stroke? Neurorehabilitation and Neural Repair 23, 313–319.

Luke, L.M., Allred, R.P., Jones, T.A., 2004. Unilateral ischemic sensorimotor cortical damage induces contralesional synaptogenesis and enhances skilled reaching with the ipsilateral forelimb in adult male rats. Synapse. 54, 187–199.

Lundy-Ekman, L., 2009. Neuroscience: fundamentals for rehabilitation WB Saunders.

Madhavan, S., Rogers, L.M., Stinear, J.W., 2010. A paradox: after stroke, the non-lesioned lower limb motor cortex may be maladaptive. European Journal of Neuroscience 32, 1032–1039.

Markus, T.M., Tsai, S.Y., Bollnow, M.R., et al., 2005. Recovery and brain reorganization after stroke in adult and aged rats. Annals of Neurology 58, 950–953.

Mcdonnell, M.N., Koblar, S., Ward, N.S., et al., 2015. An investigation of cortical neuroplasticity following stroke in adults: is there evidence for a critical window for rehabilitation? BMC Neurology 15.

Merzenich, M.M., Nelson, R.J., Stryker, M.P., 1984. Somatosensory cortical map changes following digit amputation in adult monkeys. Journal of Comparative Neurology 224, 591–605.

Monfils, M.H., Teskey, G.C., 2004. Skilled-learning-induced potentiation in rat sensorimotor cortex: a transient form of behavioural long-term potentiation. Neuroscience. 125, 329–336.

Morton, S.M., Bastian, A.J., 2007. Mechanisms of cerebellar gait ataxia. Cerebellum. 6, 79–86.

Nambu, A., Tokuno, H., Takada, M., 2002. Functional significance of the cortico–subthalamo–pallidal 'hyperdirect' pathway. Neuroscience Research 43, 111–117.

Nielsen, J.B., 2003. How we walk: central control of muscle activity during human walking. Neuroscientist. 9, 195–204.

Nithianantharajah, J., Hannan, A.J., 2006. Enriched environments, experience-dependent plasticity and disorders of the nervous system. Nature Reviews Neuroscience 7, 697–709.

Nudo, R.J., 2013. Recovery after brain injury: mechanisms and principles. Frontiers in Human Neuroscience 7, 887.

Nudo, R.J., Milliken, G.W., Jenkins, W.M., Merzenich, M.M., 1996. Use-dependent alterations of movement representations in primary motor cortex of adult squirrel monkeys. Journal of Neuroscience 16, 785–807.

Plautz, E.J., Milliken, G.W., Nudo, R.J., 2000. Effects of repetitive motor training on movement representations in adult squirrel monkeys: role of use versus learning. Neurobiology of Learning and Memory 74, 27–55.

Porter, R., Lemon, R., 1993. Corticospinal Function and Voluntary Movement. Clarendon Press, Oxford.

Rathelot, J.A., Strick, P.L., 2006. Muscle representation in the macaque motor cortex: an anatomical perspective. Proceedings of the National Academy of Sciences of the United States of America 103, 8257–8262. http://doi.org/10.1073/pnas.0602933103.

Remple, M.S., Bruneau, R.M., Vandenberg, P.M., Goertzen, C., Kleim, J.A., 2001. Sensitivity of cortical movement representations to motor experience: evidence that skill learning but not strength training induces cortical reorganization. Behavioural Brain Research 123, 133–141.

Rizzolatti, G., Fadiga, L., Gallese, V., Fogassi, L., 1996. Premotor cortex and the recognition of motor actions. Brain Research. Cognitive Brain Research 3, 131–141.

Rosenzweig, E.S., Brock, J.H., Culbertson, M.D., et al., 2009. Extensive spinal decussation and bilateral termination of cervical corticospinal projections in rhesus monkeys. The Journal of Comparative Neurology 513, 151–163.

Sale, M.V., Ridding, M.C., Nordstrom, M.A., 2008. Cortisol inhibits neuroplasticity induction in human motor cortex. Journal of Neuroscience 28, 8285–8293.

Schmidt, R., Lee, T., 2013. Motor Learning and Performance, 5E With Web Study Guide: From Principles to Application. Human Kinetics Publishers (Champaign, United States).

Shumway-Cook, A.W.M.H., 2012. Motor Control: Translating Research Into Clinical Practice. Wolters Kluwer Health/Lippincott Williams & Wilkins, Philadelphia.

Stefan, K., Wycislo, M., Classen, J., 2004. Modulation of associative human motor cortical plasticity by attention. Journal of Neurophysiology 92, 66–72.

Stinear, C.M., Barber, P.A., Petoe, M., Anwar, S., Byblow, W.D., 2012. The PREP algorithm predicts potential for upper limb recovery after stroke. Brain. 135, 2527–2535.

Stinear, C.M., Byblow, W.D., Ackerley, S.J., Barber, P.A., Smith, M.C., 2017. Predicting recovery potential for individual stroke patients increases rehabilitation efficiency. Stroke. 48, 1011–1019.

Stoykov, M.E., Madhavan, S., 2015. Motor priming in neurorehabilitation. Journal of Neurologic Physical Therapy 39, 33–42.

Todd, G., Kimber, T.E., Ridding, M.C., Semmler, J.G., 2010. Reduced motor cortex plasticity following inhibitory rTMS in older adults. Clinical Neurophysiology 121, 441–447.

Van Vliet, P.M., Wulf, G., 2006. Extrinsic feedback for motor learning after stroke: what is the evidence? Disability and Rehabilitation 28, 831–840.

Verheyden, G., Vereeck, L., Truijen, S., et al., 2006. Trunk performance after stroke and the relationship with balance, gait and functional ability. Clinical Rehabilitation 20, 451–458.

Wassermann, E., Epstein, C., Ziemann, U., et al., 2008. Oxford Handbook of Transcranial Stimulation. OUP, Oxford.

Werhahn, K.J., Mortensen, J., Kaelin-Lang, A., Boroojerdi, B., Cohen, L.G., 2002. Cortical excitability changes induced by deafferentation of the contralateral hemisphere. Brain. 125, 1402–1413.

Willerslev-Olsen, M., Lundbye-Jensen, J., Petersen, T.H., Nielsen, J.B., 2011. The effect of baclofen and diazepam on motor skill acquisition in healthy subjects. Experimental Brain Research 213, 465.

Winstein, C.J., Rose, D.K., Tan, S.M., et al., 2004. A randomized controlled comparison of upper-extremity rehabilitation strategies in acute stroke: a pilot study of immediate and long-term outcomes. Archives of Physical Medicine and Rehabilitation. 85, 620–628.

Wulf, G., 2013. Attentional focus and motor learning: a review of 15 years. International Review of Sport and Exercise Psychology 6, 77–104.

Ziemann, U., Muellbacher, W., Hallett, M., Cohen, L.G., 2001. Modulation of practice-dependent plasticity in human motor cortex. Brain. 124, 1171–1181.

CHAPTER 3

Motor training

Sheila Lennon

INTRODUCTION

The role of the physiotherapist working in neurology is to help the patient experience and relearn optimal movement and functional activity based on an understanding of how the nervous system controls movement and the application of motor learning for skill acquisition (see Chapter 1 for guiding principles in neurological rehabilitation). Motor training in neurological physiotherapy emerges from a complex clinical reasoning process derived from an understanding of optimal movement strategies employed by neurologically intact individuals (see Chapter 4 on assessment).

Specificity of training (you gain what you train) and intensity (dose) are critical. Effective motor training should focus on high-intensity and repetitive task-specific practice which targets actions that are frequently used in everyday life. The optimal intensity for training requires further investigation. In addition to targeting specific impairments, physiotherapists work mainly on the following motor tasks:

- bed mobility (rolling, sitting up, lying down, rolling over);
- standing up and sitting down;
- transfers (bed to chair and chair to bed, on and off the floor);
- balance;
- walking; and
- upper limb function.

A reminder of the key critical movements of body segments required during these functional motor tasks is presented at the end of this chapter (see Cassidy et al 2018 for a comprehensive overview of movement analysis). Examples of movement analysis and training in this chapter relate usually to stroke, but these general principles can also apply to other conditions (see evidence for condition-specific training in later chapters; see key messages in Box 3.1).

Effective motor training in neurological physiotherapy is composed of varying combinations of six components within each therapy session: alignment, postural control (balance), selective muscle activity, training of missing components (movements or task actions), task-specific practice and independent practice (see Fig. 3.1).

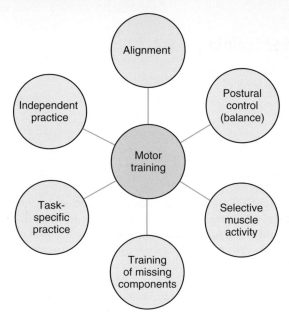

Fig. 3.1
Essential components of motor training.

Box 3.1 Training: Key Messages

● Think about the aims of physiotherapy when preparing the treatment, plan which can be summed up using the acronym RAMP (Restore, Adapt, Prevent and/or Maintain) (Lennon & Bassile 2018).
● If a patient has the potential to change, give him or her an opportunity to recover optimal movement and function rather than to use compensatory strategies which may hinder movement recovery because the patient is learning how *not* to use a limb.
● The choice of treatment strategies will depend on the patient's starting level of motor ability (Kilbride & Cassidy 2009):
   ○ No activity or minimal activity: Use gravity-eliminated exercise in the midrange or active-assisted exercise and activation of extensor activity in standing or sitting. Consider adjuncts such as electrical stimulation, biofeedback, mental practice, mirror therapy, etc.
   ○ With some activity: Focus on modified task practice and strength training.

Box 3.1 Training: Key Messages—cont'd

- Use manual assistance sparingly:
  - If the patient cannot move independently, try changing his position or assisting him to move with manual guidance to help the patient experience movement and activity.
  - Think about why you are using manual assistance: to align, to facilitate/assist movement and to block/restrict a movement (Ryerson & Levitt 1997, pp. 60–63).
  - Consider other options such as the need for support (if any), for example, parallel bars, wall or table on stronger side, walking aid or assistive technology.

ESSENTIAL COMPONENTS OF MOTOR TRAINING

- **Alignment (Shumway-Cook & Woollacott 2017, p. 158):** Biomechanical alignment of body segments requires minimal muscular effort to remain in the vertical position. Postural tone keeps the body from collapsing in response to gravity. Trunk muscle activity is critical to maintaining balance in sitting and standing. Emphasis on being upright is very important to stimulate antigravity activity and balance. Good posture provides stability for mobility (see Box 3.2).

Box 3.2 Alignment: Key Messages

- Consider alignment and symmetry for more efficient muscle activation.
- Work on lengthening and strengthening relevant muscles. Always address soft tissue changes.
- Remember that maintaining balance on any base of support is a complex functional motor goal, and its loss is neither an impairment nor an activity limitation. It is usually a result of various impairments (Ada & Canning 2009).
- Work in sitting and standing positions as soon as possible. Do not wait for recovery to occur; use manual assistance with one or two therapists if necessary.

- **Postural control (balance):** Balance is the recovery of stability after displacement which brings the centre of gravity (COG) back within the base of support (BOS), enabling the patient to maintain orientation of his or her body position and movement in space. Postural muscles are activated before voluntary movements to minimise displacements (anticipatory postural adjustments). Balance is a complex functional motor goal that requires task-specific training (see Lubetzky-Vilnai & Kartin 2010 for a systematic review for individuals poststroke). Visual, vestibular and somatosensory inputs contribute to postural control. Postural control is attentionally demanding; maintaining balance while performing another task can be detrimental to performance (see Box 3.3).

Box 3.3 Postural Control: Key Messages

- Consider how the patient is able to actively move their COG with respect to their BOS to target postural control (balance).
- Practice weight transfer (WT) using pelvic tilting to gain postural adjustments and limb loading.
- Practice maintaining the COG over the BOS, moving outside the BOS, and regaining the COG within the BOS (Shumway-Cook & Woollacott 2017, p. 155).
- Consider manipulating visual (verticality; eyes open/closed), vestibular (head position) and somatosensory systems (see Meldrum & McConn Walsh 2018).
- Balance may need to be trained first under single- and then under dual-task conditions (e.g. initially stop talking while walking).

- **Training selective control:** Lack of selective control refers to the inability to voluntarily move one body segment independently of other segments (Lang et al 2009); for example, after a stroke the patient may flex the shoulder, elbow and fingers when trying to bend their elbow. Patients attempt to achieve their motor goals using movement strategies that differ from those that would normally be used (see Box 3.4).

Box 3.4 Selective Control: Key Messages

- Compensatory (adaptive) strategies may not always represent the optimal way to perform a task.
- Patients need to be trained to use more functional patterns which allow flexibility according to the environmental features and goals of their actions (Carr & Shepherd 2010, Chapter 2).

- **Training of missing components:** When assessing and treating patients with neurological problems, physiotherapists use movement analysis to identify the critical features that are affected or missing, without which functional tasks would not be possible (Carr & Shepherd 2006). These individual movements or task components that are absent or difficult to perform can be practiced in parts before the whole task is practised. Trunk control is a critical component that is often impaired or absent in neurological patients. For example, when a patient attempts to take off his top, the trunk may be placed too far backwards in posterior pelvic tilt and the feet may leave the floor. Thus neurological therapists will work on targeting trunk control before and during upper limb movement (see Box 3.5).

Box 3.5 Trunk Control: Key Messages

- Target trunk control (Song & Heo 2015), as well as control of limbs, to train postural control, balance and limb movement and function.
- Exercises that target trunk control can improve trunk function and potentially balance, gait and mobility, with the most recent systematic review emphasising practicing on an unstable surface (Cabanas-Valdes et al 2013, Van Criekinge et al 2017):
  - Two protocols have been recommended for the trunk after a stroke: a 5-minute warm-up of loading the leg and looking behind; 20 minutes of task-specific sitting training, including reaching to the table in front of the patient with the nonaffected hand and reaching to the floor; and a 5-minute cool-down for 30 minutes per session, five times a week for 2 weeks (Ada et al 2006).
  - Selective trunk movements of the upper and lower part of the trunk in lying, include rolling, abdominal muscle activation, pelvic movement and bridging, and in sitting with selective flexion/extension, lateral flexion and rotation from the trunk, shoulder and pelvic girdle, as well as reaching (Saeys et al 2012, Verheyden et al 2009).

- **Task-specific practice:** The practice of motor skills needs to be both task and context specific (French et al 2016); for example, if the therapist wants walking to improve, the patient needs to actually practice walking! Intervention should always focus on the function and goals of the individual and not simply be aimed at improving impairments. It is always preferable to practice functional tasks; however, when the patient has impairments that make it difficult to practice the task directly, therapists will also need to address impairments, either before or during a modified version of functional task practice (Lennon & Bassile 2018; see Box 3.6).

Box 3.6 Task-specific Practice: Key Messages

- Always ask the patient to try to practice the task first; if this is unsuccessful, then consider the components of the task and the environmental setup to determine how best to modify the task for success (e.g. raise the seat height when practicing sit to stand).

● **Independent practice:** Many repetitions and hours of activity are required to regain a skill, and therapy time is limited; therefore it is essential to give the patient ways of exercising alone or under supervision or with assistance of their carers to achieve the intensity required for skill acquisition (see Box 3.7). Given the negative effects of physical inactivity and sedentary behaviour (see Dawes 2018), there are sound reasons for prescribing practice independently from dedicated therapy sessions:

   ● increasing intensity of practice;
   ● increasing consistency of practice;
   ● encouraging carry over between therapy sessions;
   ● encouraging active problem solving and self-management; and
   ● building confidence and self-efficacy.

Box 3.7 Practice: Key Messages

> ● Make sure the patient is actively involved in problem solving why he/she has movement dysfunction and understands which exercises/activities are critical to practice.
> ● Always find a way in even the most severely affected patients to enable them to practice outside dedicated therapy sessions.

CRITICAL FEATURES OF FUNCTIONAL ACTIVITIES: A REMINDER

The therapist needs to know the critical features involved in performing functional mobility tasks so that he/she can identify and train the missing components. Rolling over, lying to sitting and standing up are presented in Table 3.1. Walking components are presented in Table 3.2. Essential components of upper limb function are presented in Table 3.3.

See Cassidy et al 2018 for a comprehensive review of movement analysis.

Table 3.1 Key movements for analysis of rolling over, lying to sitting, and standing up (based on Carr & Shepherd 2010)

Activity	Head	Trunk/pelvis	Upper limb	Lower limb
Rolling to one side	Flexes and rotates towards turning side	Rotation	Shoulder protraction and flexion	Upper leg, hip and knee flex over the weight-bearing (WB) side
Side-lying to sitting	Side flexes	WB side elongates Upper side laterally flexes	Abduction of the WB arm	Legs are lifted and swung over the side
Sitting to standing	Extends	Inclination of the extended trunk forward Pelvis moves into anterior tilt	Arms vary	Foot placement Feet move backwards into dorsiflexion (ankles behind knees) Knees move forward over feet Hips and knees extend for final alignment

Table 3.2 Critical features and kinematics of walking (based on Cassidy et al 2018)

Stance phase (60% of the cycle)	Critical features (Carr & Shepherd 2010)
The lower limb extensors and bio-mechanical alignment bear the weight and prevent the limb from collapsing	● Hip extension with dorsiflexion. ● Lateral pelvic shift to stance side. ● Fifteen degrees of knee flexion at initial contact to load the limb, followed by extension in midstance, then flexion before push-off. ● Plantarflexion at initial contact followed by dorsiflexion then plantarflexion for push-off.
	Kinematics (Whittle et al 2012)
From initial contact (IC) to loading response (LR) Aim: Weight acceptance	● The hip moves into extension. ● The knee moves from extension to slight knee flexion by eccentric contraction of the quadriceps. ● The ankle moves into plantarflexion through the eccentric action of the tibialis anterior to bring the forefoot in contact with the ground.

continued

Table 3.2 Critical features and kinematics of walking (based on Cassidy et al 2018)—cont'd

Stance phase (60% of the cycle)	Critical features (Carr & Shepherd 2010)
LR to midstance (MST) Aim: Weight-bearing to prevent limb collapse	• The hip continues to extend through gravity and inertia. • Weight transfer occurs by lateral pelvic horizontal movement towards the stance leg controlled by the hip abductors. • The knee extends through concentric action of the quadriceps. • The tibia moves forward over the foot through the eccentric action of the plantar flexors.
Terminal stance (TST) Aim: Preparation for swing	• The hip reaches maximum extension (10–20 degrees) just as the opposite leg achieves initial contact. The abductors stabilise the pelvis. • The knee begins to flex. • The ankle moves into plantarflexion.
Preswing (PS) Aim: Push-off	• Hip flexion is initiated in preparation to swing the leg forward. • The knee moves rapidly into flexion controlled by eccentric contraction of the rectus femoris in preparation for toe clearance. • The ankle continues to move into plantarflexion through the concentric action of the plantar flexors. • The toes extend at the metatarsophalangeal joints.
Swing phase (40% of the cycle)	**Critical features (Carr & Shepherd 2010)**
Aim: Foot clearance for accurate and safe foot placement at initial contact	• Hip flexion. • Knee flexion with lateral pelvic tilt towards the swing side. • Rotation of the pelvis forward on the swing side. • Knee extension plus ankle dorsiflexion for toe clearance.
	Kinematics (Whittle et al 2012)
	• The hip continues to flex. • The knee continues to flex to shorten the leg, then swings into extension. • The tibialis anterior contracts during mid-swing to dorsiflex the foot during the rest of the swing.

Upper limb function involves: grasping and releasing objects; transporting objects from one place to another; manipulating objects for specific purposes; reaching in all directions, and using both hands together, or independently (Carr & Shepherd 2010).

Table 3.3 Essential components of reaching and manipulation (based on McCluskey et al 2017)

Reaching	● Shoulder flexion, abduction, extension depending on direction of reach (Carr & Shepherd 2010) ● Scapular protraction (Yang et al 2014) ● Elbow extension with varying amounts of external shoulder rotation ● Pronation and supination appropriate to object orientation
Preshaping	● Ulnar or radial deviation ● Supination ● Wrist extension ● Thumb abduction ● Thumb opposition ● Metacarpophalangeal extension ● Interphalangeal flexion ● Finger abduction
Object grasp and release Power grip (the fingers and thumb are directed towards the palm) Precision grip (forces are directed between the thumb and the fingers)	● Extension of the wrist and fingers with radial deviation for optimal hand opening ● Extension and opposition of the thumb to the fifth finger (Lang et al 2009) ● Thumb adduction and flexion with interphalangeal flexion for closure of the fingers and thumb around an object
Object manipulation and finger dexterity	● Independent finger flexion and extension (e.g. tapping) ● Abduction and opposition of the thumb to the fifth finger (e.g. cupping) ● Holding, placing and rotating objects with supination and pronation

References

Ada, L., Dean, C.M., Mackey, F., 2006. Increasing the amount of physical activity undertaken after stroke. Physical Therapy Review 11, 91–100.

Ada, L., Canning, C., 2009. Common motor impairments and their impact on activity. In: Lennon, S., Stokes, M. (Eds.), Pocketbook of Neurological Physiotherapy. Elsevier Science, London.

Cabanas-Valdés, R., Cuchi, G.U., Bagur-Calafat, C., 2013. Trunk training exercises approaches for improving trunk performance and functional sitting balance in patients with stroke: a systematic review. Neurorehabilitation 33, 575–592.

Carr, J.H., Shepherd, R.B., 2006. Neurological rehabilitation. Disability & Rehabilitation 28, 811–812.

Carr, J.H., Shepherd, R.B., 2010. Neurological rehabilitation: optimising motor performance, third ed. Butterworth Heinemann, Oxford.

Cassidy, E., Wallace, A., Bunn, L., 2018. Observation and analysis of movement. In: Lennon, S., Ramdharry, G., Verheyden, G. (Eds.), Physical Management for Neurological Conditions, fourth ed. Elsevier, London.

Dawes, H., 2018. Physical activity and exercise. In: Lennon, S., Ramdharry, G., Verheyden, G. (Eds.), Physical Management for Neurological Conditions, fourth ed. Elsevier, London.

French, B., Thomas, L.H., Coupe, J., McMahon, N.E., Connell, L., Harrison, J., et al., 2016. Repetitive task training for improving functional ability after stroke. Cochrane Database of Systematic Reviews 11, CD006073.

Kilbride, C., Cassidy, E., 2009. The stable acute patient with potential for recovery: stroke, brain injury, Guillain Barré Syndrome. In: Lennon, S., Stokes, M. (Eds.), Pocketbook of Neurological Physiotherapy. Elsevier Science, London.

Lang, C.E., DE Jong, S., Beebe, J.A., 2009. Recovery of thumb extension and its relation to grasp performance after stroke. Journal of Physiology 102, 451–459.

Lennon, S., Bassile, C., 2018. Guiding principles in neurological rehabilitation. In: Lennon, S., Ramdharry, G., Verheyden, G. (Eds.), Physical Management for Neurological Conditions, fourth ed. Elsevier, London.

Lubetzky-Vilnai, A., Kartin, D., 2010. The effect of balance training on balance performance in individuals post stroke: a systematic review. Journal of Neurologic Physical Therapy 34, 127–137.

McCluskey, A., Lannin, N.A., Schurr, K., Dorsch, S., 2017. Optimisimg motor performance and sensation after brain impairment. In: Curtin, M., Egan, M., Adams, E. (Eds.), Occupational Therapy for people experiencing illness, injury or impairment: promoting occupation and participation, seventh ed. Elsevier, Australia.

Meldrum D, McConn Walsh. Vestibular Rehabilitation. In: Lennon, S., Ramdharry, G., Verheyden, G. (Eds.), Physical Management for Neurological Conditions, fourth ed. Elsevier, London.

Ryerson, S., Levit, K., 1997. Functional Movement Reeducation. Churchill Livingstone, Edinburgh.

Saeys, W., Vereeck, L., Truijen, S., Lafosse, C., Wuyts, F.P., Van de Heyning, P., 2012. Randomized controlled trial of truncal exercises early after stroke to improve balance and mobility. Neurorehabilitation and Neural Repair 26, 231–238.

Shumway-Cook, A., Woollacott, M.H., 2017. Motor control translating research into clinical practice, fifth ed. Williams & Wilkins, Baltimore.

Song, G., Heo, J.Y., 2015. The effect of modified bridging exercise on the balance ability of stroke patients. Journal of Physical Therapy Science 27 (12), 3807–3810.

Van Criekinge, T., Saeys, W., Vereeck, L., De Hertogh, W., Truijen, S., 2017. Are unstable support surfaces superior to stable support surfaces during trunk rehabilitation after stroke? A systematic review. Disability & Rehabilitation 39, 1–8.

Verheyden, G., Vereeck, L., Truijen, S., Troch, M., Lafosse, C., Saeys, W., DeWeerdt, W., 2009. Additional exercises improve trunk performance after stroke: a pilot randomized controlled trial. Neurorehabilitation and Neural Repair 23 (3), 281–286.

Whittle, M.W., Levine, D., Richards, J., 2012. Normal gait. In: Levine, D., Richards, J., Whittle, M.W. (Eds.), Whittle's Gait Analysis: an introduction, fifth ed. Churchill Livingstone, Elsevier, Edinburgh.

Yang, J., Lee, J., Lee, B., Jeon, S., et al., 2014. The effects of active scapular protraction on the muscle activation and function of the upper extremity. Journal of Physical Therapy Science 26, 599–603.

CHAPTER 4

Neurological assessment: the basis of clinical decision making

Jill Garner and Sheila Lennon

INTRODUCTION

Physiotherapists use the process of clinical reasoning combined with current evidence and the patient/family perspective to assess, develop and evaluate an appropriate plan of care for each patient (World Confederation for Physical Therapy [WCPT] 2011a).

Assessment is always the starting point for clinical reasoning. It is based on the International Classification of Functioning, Disability and Health (ICF) framework for rehabilitation (Fig. 4.1), where the therapist identifies underlying impairments, activity limitations and participation restrictions (World Health Organization [WHO] 2001).

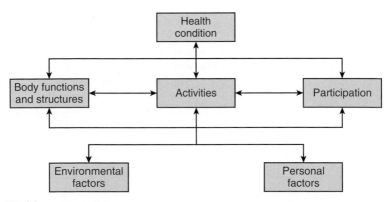

Fig. 4.1
The ICF (WHO 2001).

A comprehensive assessment (Bland et al 2015):
- facilitates decision making and treatment planning;
- helps determine patient prognosis;

- helps therapists select appropriate interventions; and
- helps therapists consider the need for additional services.

There is no standardised process for neurological assessment. Assessment components will vary according to the condition, the type of setting, prognosis and the reasons for referral to physiotherapy.

Assessment consists of two parts: a subjective exploration of the person's perspective of an issue and an objective examination of performance. The objective assessment includes observation, physical examination and the use of standardised measurement tools with published reliability and validity (Table 4.1).

Table 4.1 Key elements of an assessment

Subjective	Objective
● Information gathering from the patient's medical record/chart	● Observation
● Liaison with the care team	● Examination
● Interviewing the patient/family	● Standardised measurement tools

Why Assess?

Assessment establishes a baseline of a patient's status at a specific point in time. This enables the therapist to decide what he or she can affect and in what way. During the assessment the therapist will consider other factors that may have an impact on assessment or treatment.

A therapist's communication style is important to establish rapport with the patient. You are aiming to gradually uncover the patient's perception of their issues; this may take time. Generally, throughout the assessment note the patient's:

- ability to follow instructions,
- mental state/mood and behaviour, especially highlighting anxiety, emotional lability, depression and/or aggression; and
- wishes and choices.

Tips for communication with patients with neurological problems:
- Simplify your questions.
- If speech is impaired, ask yes and no questions (see speech pathology report).
- Give the patient more time to answer.
- Use gestures.
- Change voice volume or speed of talking.
- Ask a carer or family member for clarification.

HOW TO COMPLETE A NEUROLOGICAL ASSESSMENT
Is Your Patient Medically Stable?

Always start by reviewing the patient's medical record and confirm that the patient is medically stable by liaising with the care team and checking vital signs. Acute patients may be unstable; the physiotherapist must monitor vital signs carefully before assessing or treating patients.

Use the data obtained from the medical record (Box 4.1) and team consultation to decide if you are going to assess in situ or change the patient's position. In the acute stage, it is often better to schedule shorter, more frequent sessions.

Physiotherapy applied inappropriately when the patient is unstable may make the patient worse – for example, deciding to sit a patient up out of bed, when his or her blood pressure is too low.

Box 4.1 Key Database Information

Diagnosis
Date of onset
Investigations
● Cardiovascular stability: BP, HR, RR, ECG
● ABGs
● FBC (HGB; WBC)
● Scan
● X-rays

BP, Blood pressure; *HR*, heart rate; *RR*, respiratory rate; *ABG*, arterial blood gas; *FBC*, full blood count; *HGB*, haemoglobin; *WBC*, white blood cells.

Remember that patients with neurological conditions may also be ventilated, paralysed and sedated with impaired levels of consciousness (LOC) during the acute phase. You do not need to wait for the patient to wake up or move spontaneously before assessing them. However, at this stage, you may need to keep change of positions to a minimum. Sessions may need to be shorter and more frequent. (Kilbride & Cassidy 2009a).

In patients with an impaired LOC:

● Never talk over a patient; always assume they can hear you and understand what you are saying.
● Modify the environment by pulling the curtains around the bed to minimise distractions.
● Aim to reduce noise levels

4

Kilbride and Cassidy (2009b) recommend you ask yourself the following key questions before you physically assess a patient:

● Do I need to move the patient, or can I start my assessment in situ? A change of posture may adversely affect patient stability and can be unnecessarily fatiguing.
● What can the patient do by themselves? Encourage active participation whenever possible.
● If the patient is unable to move independently, does changing the patient's position wake them up and help them move?

Subjective Assessment

The next step is to interview the patient and/or family caregiver to record the subjective information:

● Make sure you introduce yourself and gain consent for assessment.
● Check you are assessing the correct patient using three patient identifiers: name, date of birth and medical record number/address (O'Rourke 2007).

During the interview, you are aiming to find out about the patient's current symptoms and their understanding of why they have been admitted to hospital or referred for physiotherapy; past medical history; and social history that involves family, work, hobbies and accommodation, as well as to gain an idea of their general mobility and function (Box 4.2).

Box 4.2 Subjective Assessment

> **HPC (History of the Present Condition):** Tell me why you are here. What problems are bothering you?
> ● You may need to ask your patient if they have noticed any issues with speech or swallowing; hearing or changes to vision, continence, fatigue or pain.
> **PMH (Past Medical History):** Check the main points from the record, or delve deeper during the interview if there is not enough information.
> **SOCIAL SITUATION:**
> **Work:** Before this incident/episode, were you working? If so what did this involve?
> **Hobbies:** What do you do in your spare time? In your average day what do you spend your time doing?
> **Family:** Tell me about your living situation. Do you live alone or have someone at home with you? Do they support you in any way? Do you receive support from friends or other family members?

Box 4.2 Subjective Assessment—cont'd

Home: Do you have any steps to access your home or any stairs inside? If so, where are they? How many? Are there any rails? Has your home been modified in any way to assist you or others to live in it?

Other services: Do you receive any external support from other agencies such as the council, private agencies or others? How often does this happen, and what time of day does this occur?

Access to the community: How do you get out and about? This question may involve previous and current ability to drive.

GENERAL MOBILITY LEVEL:

Before this incident/episode, were you using a walking aid? If so, for how long and who gave this to you? How far do you usually walk a day, and how long would this take you? Do you do any other exercises, whether formal or informal?

Or

Since this episode, what are you able to do for yourself? (The patient may need prompting to talk about functional mobility and self-care.)

PATIENT'S EXPRESSED GOALS/EXPECTATIONS:

What would you like to work on or focus on during therapy or while you're here in hospital?

GENERAL OBSERVATIONS:

If sitting or lying, observe posture (noting symmetry), spontaneous ability to move
If walking into the consulting room, note gait.

MENTAL STATE:

Mood and manner in which the patient answers questions. Check orientation to time, person and place, as required.

COMMUNICATION:

Note dysarthria, expressive or receptive dysphasia during questioning.

FALLS HISTORY (If the client has a chronic neurological disorder or is > 65 years): Have you had any recent falls? Tell me what happened? How many and over what time period? Have you had some near falls when you have not hit the floor? Tell me about them.

The Objective Examination

Observation is an important assessment skill for any physiotherapist (Box 4.3):

● Get prepared for the physical examination.
● Check the environment and plan for what you may need (e.g. space to manoeuvre, a chair, a walking aid or physical assistance/standby of one or two people).
● Start by explaining what you are going to do and why, while you are observing your patient.

Box 4.3 Observation

- Observe the patient's posture and alignment of the head, the trunk and the limbs.
- Consider the need to use demonstration to show the patient what you want them to do.
- Ask the patient to show you how they can move independently.
- If the patient can move, is it effortful, easy, smooth or uncoordinated?
- Compare the patient's movements to key features derived from normal movement performance (see Carr & Shepherd 2010, Cassidy et al 2018)
- Look out for compensations.
- If the patient cannot move, does assisting the patient to move and/or changing his or her position improve patient performance?

During the objective examination:

- Start by assessing the patient in the position you find them in.

  You may need to change the order of assessment depending on whether the patient walks in or is in a chair or the bed.

  If the patient is sitting, you should assess volitional movement and strength (limbs) and balance (trunk), as well as the ability to stand, before attempting to transfer the patient to the treatment plinth.

- Consider manual handling risk assessment.

  Do a risk assessment before transferring a patient. Legislation varies across countries; however, a simple way to remember what to think about is to use the acronym TILE: the Task, the Individual, the Load (can the patient assist you?) and the Environment (Chartered Society of Physiotherapy 2014). Annual training/review in manual handling is usually required to maintain knowledge and skills.

- Identify if there are postural control and movement deficits (alignment and weight transference ability) and other neurological impairments which affect the patient's ability to move and function.

- Assess the patient's functional level, noting the activities the patient is able to perform independently in an optimal manner with or without compensatory patterns. Consider nighttime versus daytime function.

- Be careful when cueing during the assessment – the functional task is only independent without any verbal or manual cues.

- Therapeutic handling (manual assistance).

  - Do not physically assist the patient unless safety is a concern; always ask a patient to show you how they can move independently first, but stand close enough that you can intervene as necessary.

● Note the aim of therapeutic handling (manual assistance) is to produce new movement or allow a previously impossible activity to be performed. Physical assistance may be used to correct alignment, to limit degrees of freedom of a joint, to block unwanted movement or to stabilise a weak joint or body segment (Ryerson & Levit 1997).

The Physical Examination

Although it is essential to assess range, weakness and functional performance similar to any other type of assessment, several impairments are unique and important in neurological assessment (see McLoughlin 2018 for a review of common impairments in neurology and their impact on activity). The key components of the examination are presented in Table 4.2. A blank sample assessment form is presented in Table 4.3 (from Ryerson 2009 with permission).

Table 4.2 Key components of the physical examination

Chest status Swallowing/ feeding	With recent episode of deterioration or during an acute admission: ● Note increased temperature. ● Perform chest assessment to determine respiratory status and need for chest treatment. ● Check ability to cough. ● Check swallowing or speech problems.
Cranial nerve assessment	● Cranial nerve assessment is especially important in medullary stroke. Usually performed by the neurologist and can be obtained from the medical record.

Vision	● Visual testing allows the therapist to ascertain if the patient can see their entire environment and indicate to the therapist where best to position themselves to facilitate visual scanning and/or so the patient can see the therapist during therapy sessions.
	● Visual fields
	  ● Start with the fingers just in front of the ears – need to test 360 degrees, with patient looking at the therapist's nose so they see the therapist's fingers; do randomly, one side at a time.
	  ● Keep looking at my nose; is my finger moving? Or how many fingers can you see?
	  ● Assess eye range of movement and if the patient can keep their eyes focused on your finger or pen and follow it when moved (smooth pursuit 20 degrees per second).
	  ● To test, hold finger/pen arm's length away from client – 'Look at the tip of my finger', or tip of my pen, hold chin lightly.
	  ● Move pen 20–30 degrees horizontally and then vertically.
	● Perform full oculomotor examination if patient reports symptoms of dizziness or vertiginous symptoms to identify if cause of problem is central and/or peripheral.

continued

Table 4.2 Key components of the physical examination—cont'd

Head and trunk activity	<ul><li>Note position of head when moving from one posture to another.</li><li>Note ability to right head to midline after dynamic activities.</li><li>Note resting posture: symmetrical or asymmetrical?</li><li>Pelvic tilting is our main mechanism of weight transfer. Ability to pelvic tilt – anterior/posterior tilt versus lateral tilt. Lateral tilt – check for elongation over weight-bearing (WB) side and side flexion on non-WB side.</li></ul>
Sitting balance	Postural control is assessed statically and dynamically.<ul><li>Static: To determine the ability to stay upright over the base of support and withstand the force of gravity.</li><li>Dynamic: To assess the ability of the body to remain upright during movement of the limbs, head and eyes outside the base of support and the ability of the body to respond to external environmental perturbations and cognitive distraction.</li><li>Is the patient able to sit independently and symmetrically without using their arms for balance?</li><li>Attempt reaching out of the base of support: Note elongation over WB side when reaching and the ability to return to midline.</li></ul>
Reflexes	<ul><li>Presence or absence of deep tendon reflexes helps identify lower motor neurone issues.</li><li>Hyperactive reflexes are indicative of abnormal tone.</li></ul>
Upper limb (posture/ROM/tone/altered volitional movement/strength) Shoulder Elbow Wrist and hand	<ul><li>Pain in shoulder may limit ability to perform passive range of motion (PROM). Compare to less affected side.</li><li>Tone: Test by resistance to passive stretching. Test for spasticity through quick stretch of muscle. Note contractures or any pain associated with testing.</li><li>Altered volitional movement: Impaired selective movement which refers to the ability to initiate, sustain, cease and sequence movement patterns.</li><li>Loss of selective muscle activation and abnormal synergies (Shumway-Cook & Woollacott 2017, pp. 111–112).</li><li>Strength: Manual muscle testing of major muscle groups.</li><li>Function of upper limb: Ability to perform functional tasks such as bringing a cup to the mouth.</li><li>Note any involuntary movements such as dyskinesia or dystonia.</li></ul>
Lower limbs (posture/ROM/tone/altered volitional movement/strength) Hip Knee Foot and ankle	<ul><li>Compare to less affected side: active range of motion (AROM), PROM.</li><li>Tone: Test by resistance to passive stretching. Test for spasticity through quick stretch of muscle, commonly quads, hamstring, tibialis anterior, tibialis posterior, gastrocnemius, soleus; note contracture of joints, any pain or involuntary movements.</li><li>Altered volitional movement: Impaired selective movement, which refers to the ability to initiate, sustain, cease and sequence movement patterns.</li><li>Loss of selective muscle activation and abnormal synergies (Shumway-Cook & Woollacott 2017, pp. 111–112).</li></ul>

Table 4.2 Key components of the physical examination—cont'd

Sensation	Light touch (eyes closed) ● Use cotton wool. 'Tell me where and when I am touching you'. Touch generally shoulder, forearm and hand. Temperature testing (comparing sides): Use test tubes with hot and cold water. Proprioception (joint position sense = JPS) ● Start with distal joint, then test proximally if fine JPS is impaired. ● For gross JPS, use mirror image with therapist placing the affected arm and patient demonstrating the position with the less affected arm. ● Score the number correct over the number of attempts.
Coordination	Finger–nose test ● Hold your finger about 1 meter away and ask the patient to touch your finger and back again; perform in sitting position. Heel–shin test ● Ask patient to perform on less affected side first by placing the heel on the opposite shin and sliding it down to the ankle. ● Should be accurate and not ataxic; perform this in lying position. Diadochokinesis: Rapidly alternating movement. ● For the upper limb (UL) place both hands on lap or one hand on top of the other. ● For the lower limb (LL) foot tapping, need feet a little forward in sitting so foot not in inner range of dorsiflexion.
Functional mobility Rolling over in bed Lying to sitting Sit to stand	● Compare the patient's performance to normal performance, and identify the key missing or impaired components in each functional task (see Carr & Shepherd 2010, Cassidy et al 2018). ● Before moving between positions, set up the environment to allow enough space to perform the functional task safely. ● Assistance may be needed with initiation of movement (e.g. cues to complete the movement, breaking down into steps, support/bracing of all or part of a limb or trunk). ● Demonstration of the task may be required. ● If safe to do so, allow the patient to show you how they usually perform the task. ● Consider how the patient is performing the task. ● Are they using compensation strategies? ● What is stopping them from performing the task normally (e.g. pain, sensory changes, weakness, lack of ROM, contracture, tonal changes, etc.)?

continued

Table 4.2 Key components of the physical examination—cont'd

Transfers Chair to bed	Assess transfer ability. This will depend on UL strength, LL strength, trunk strength, head position and midline awareness and their ability to initiate. ● Hoist – for patients who have no sitting balance stand lifter; for some lower limb activity slide board transfer, stand and step, block transfer. ● If transferring to and from a wheelchair, do the brakes work on the wheelchair? Is the cushion adequate? Are the tyres fully inflated? A full wheelchair assessment can be performed at a later date if there are issues.
Standing balance	Perform this test with client barefoot; may need to compare with and without shoes. ● Note type of footwear and degree of wear. ● Observe for symmetry. ● Can the patient stand without touching or supervision from the therapist? ● Observe the patient's ability to transfer weight from leg to leg. ● Perform stepping with each foot.
Gait	● Assess suitability of walking aids used. ● If using orthotics, note type and purpose. ● Observe gait pattern from bottom up or top down. ● Review one leg cycle at a time (i.e. full gait cycle of right leg). Stance ● Consider weight transfer (WT) onto affected leg; extension of affected hip on weight bearing; heel strike at initial contact; knee control in midstance. ● WT side to side. ● WT in a step position forwards onto affected leg (weaker leg), then backwards. Swing phase ● Standing on unaffected leg. Swing through of affected leg with hip flexion, knee extension and dorsiflexion. Note: ● Distance walked. ● Level of assistance required. ● Setting (indoors, outdoors, on flat even surface, on carpet). ● Speed. ● Turning ability (speed and how many steps in both directions). ● Use of walking aids. ● Ability to be distracted and maintain gait parameters. Can patient walk and talk at the same time? ● Consider vision and perception. Further assessment may involve differing surfaces, stairs, running and ability to get on and off the floor.

Table 4.3 Physiotherapy assessment form (adapted from Ryerson 2009 with permission)

Name:	D.O.B:	
Hospital number:	Age:	
Address:	Tel No:	
Physician name & address:		
Date of hospital admission:	Date of assessment:	
Diagnosis:	Date of Onset:	
Therapist's name:	Signature:	
HISTORY OF THE PRESENT COMPLAINT (HPC) RELEVANT PAST MEDICAL HISTORY (PMH)		
SOCIAL HISTORY (SH)		
MOBILITY STATUS		
PREVIOUS MOBILITY		
PATIENT'S EXPRESSED GOALS/EXPECTATIONS GENERAL OBSERVATIONS		
MENTAL STATE COMMUNICATION		
OROFACIAL FUNCTION CHEST STATUS		
VISION	HEARING	SWALLOWING/FEEDING
SENSATION/PERCEPTION		
TONE		
SELECTIVE MOVEMENT/ROM/STRENGTH		
Head/trunk/pelvis		
Upper limbs		
Lower limbs		
BALANCE		
Static		
Dynamic		
GAIT Stance phase Swing phase		

continued

Table 4.3 Physiotherapy assessment form (adapted from Ryerson 2009 with permission)—cont'd

FUNCTIONAL MOBILITY
In/out of bed:
Lying to sitting:
Sitting to standing:
Stairs/curbs:
Transfers:

Using Standardised Measurement Tools

Measurement is a core component of physical therapy practice (WCPTa, 2011). Measurement tools can be used for (Fulk & Field-Fote 2011):

- diagnosis;
- prognosis;
- care planning;
- assessing patient progress; and
- evaluating the effectiveness of interventions.

Objective measures can inform treatment planning and decision making by enabling members of the health care team to identify and define goals, develop treatment plans and effectively monitor progress (Tyson et al 2015). Standardised measures should be used to establish a baseline of performance before physiotherapy, then at key strategic points to further document any change (see Verheyden & Tyson 2018 for further reading on measurement tools; see online sources in Box 4.4).

Remember that not everything can be measured (Lennon 1995):

1. Decide what to measure.
2. Select the best-fit measure with published reliability and validity.
3. Do not invent your own measures!
4. Choose a measure that matters to the patient.
5. Choose a measure that reflects the aim of therapy so that the effectiveness of therapy can be measured.
6. One measure is not usually enough; select a range of measures that match the different levels of the ICF.

Therapists need to use a selection of measurement tools that will evaluate if improvements in impairments and function (activity) translate into improved participation, such as quality of life and improved health status.

Box 4.4 Online sources of standardised measurement tools from Verheyden and Tyson (2018) with permission

- Recommendations for stroke, multiple sclerosis, traumatic brain injury, spinal cord injury, Parkinson disease and vestibular disorders. http://www.neuropt.org/professional-resources/neurology-section-outcome-measures-recommendations
- University of South Australia, International Centre for Allied Health Evidence: http://www.unisa.edu.au/Research/Sansom-Institute-for-Health-Research/Research/Allied-Health-Evidence/Resources/OC/ Includes neurological measurement tools (besides other domains) and some standardised instruction videos.
- Stroke-specific databases: Evidence-based review of stroke rehabilitation: http://www.ebrsr.com/evidence-review/20-outcome-measures-stroke-rehabilitation; and StrokeEngine: http://www.strokengine.ca/find-assessment/

INTERPRETING THE ASSESSMENT

Clinical decision making is the overall process of gathering and analysing assessment information. Therapists analyse the results of the assessment to come up with an hypothesis of how impairments affect movement dysfunction, function (activity) and participation (Sullivan et al 2004). The assessment process is used to guide intervention by identifying clinical problems. The therapist together with the patient and his or her family agree to joint treatment goals before collaboratively devising a treatment plan. The therapist then implements the plan and conducts periodic reassessments to evaluate the effectiveness of treatment to decide to continue with treatment or to discharge the patient (Fig. 4.2).

When developing an hypothesis to explain the problems the patient is experiencing with movement and functional activities, the therapist needs to analyse multiple variables contributing to patient performance (see Schenkman et al 2006 for further reading on Hypothesis-Oriented Algorithms for Clinicians – HOAC II).

The Problem List

A problem list is not a list of every impairment noted in the assessment; rather, the therapist develops an hypothesis based on the relevant impairments linked to the appropriate activity limitations that will become the focus of goal-setting and rehabilitation intervention strategies to improve motor performance (Shumway-Cook & Woollacott 2017, p. 142).

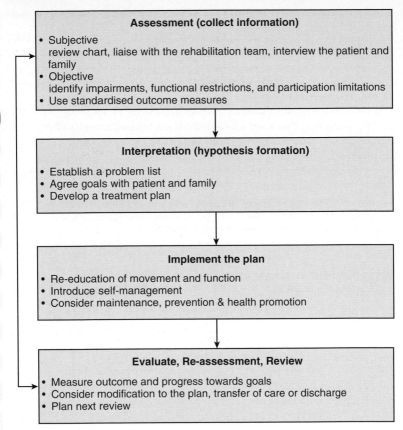

Assessment (collect information)
- Subjective
  review chart, liaise with the rehabilitation team, interview the patient and family
- Objective
  identify impairments, functional restrictions, and participation limitations
- Use standardised outcome measures

Interpretation (hypothesis formation)
- Establish a problem list
- Agree goals with patient and family
- Develop a treatment plan

Implement the plan
- Re-education of movement and function
- Introduce self-management
- Consider maintenance, prevention & health promotion

Evaluate, Re-assessment, Review
- Measure outcome and progress towards goals
- Consider modification to the plan, transfer of care or discharge
- Plan next review

Fig. 4.2
Clinical reasoning in neurological rehabilitation.

Collaborative Goal Setting

Developing an appropriate plan of care revolves around collaborative goal setting with the patient and/or the caregiver as well as the rehabilitation team (see Levack 2018 for a review of goal planning). Goals need to be based on the patient's wishes, expectations, priorities and values; one way of facilitating appropriate goal planning is to use the SMART acronym, which recommends that goals should be specific, measurable, achievable/ambitious, relevant and timed (Playford et al 2009; see Bovend'Eerdt et al 2009 for some practical guidance on how to set SMART goals).

Box 4.5 Goal setting questions from Levack (2018) with permission

- What do you hope to get out of rehabilitation?
- Where do you see yourself in 1 month? In 1 year?
- What can't you do now that you want to be able to do?
- Before your injury/illness, what was a typical day like for you? What did you do?
- Tell me about your home? What is it like? Who lives there with you?
- Tell me about your work/hobbies? What are your responsibilities? What do you do?
- What can I help you with?
- What are your main strengths? What's going to most help you through your recovery?
- What's most important to you in your life now? What do you need to be able to do to achieve this/have this?
- Tell me what you know about your current health/illness/injury.
- Do you have any concerns about your recovery that you have not talked to anyone about yet?

Tips for goal setting:
- Terminology matters!
- The patient's long-term goals are often nonspecific; you may need to ask by using a few different terms (see sample questions in Box 4.5).
- Consider organisational constraints/directives such as targets of length of stay in hospital.
- Having a goal is insufficient to create change; actions are also required.

Developing a Treatment Plan

A structured treatment plan is essential to provide appropriate interventions, which should be based on the best available evidence. It is good practice to complete a clinical reasoning form. This form enables the therapist to sum up his or her thinking (see an example of a clinical reasoning form presented later in the case scenario).

Tips for developing a treatment plan:
- Consider your patient's signs and symptoms in the context of relevant anatomy and physiology (e.g. in terms of the ascending/descending pathways affected).
- Develop an hypothesis of how impairments affect function (activity) and participation for the patient's problems.
- Form a plan from your assessment collaboratively with your patient.

- Consider possible treatment options and time frames available in each setting (e.g. acute, rehabilitation and outpatient settings).
- Use the prediction literature about recovery or disease progression to inform your patient expectations and guide your choice of interventions (Kimberley et al 2017).
- Communicate closely with the caregivers and other members of the rehabilitation team.

Implementing the Treatment Plan

Neurological physiotherapy aims to optimise movement and function with an emphasis on training control of muscles and movement and promoting learning of relevant actions and tasks to enable patients to participate in their desired life roles (Lennon & Bassile 2018).

The physiotherapist's role is to:
- reeducate movement and function;
- inform and educate;
- advise;
- support patients and their families; and
- liaise with the health care team.

Tips for delivering interventions:
- What are you aiming for in terms of RAMP (Fig. 4.3)?

  Recovery: Interventions aimed at recovery need to be emphasised over compensation if the patient has the potential to change.

  Adaptation: Focus on promoting compensatory strategies that are necessary for function and discourage those that may be detrimental to the patient (Levin et al 2009).

  Maintenance: Maintenance of function despite deteriorating impairments should be viewed as a positive achievement.

  Prevention: Consider how you can prevent the development of complications such as contracture, swelling and disuse atrophy.

- Neural plasticity is the rationale for physiotherapy intervention. The structure and the function of the nervous system can be changed through use, experience and therapy.
- Teach your patients that you are not just doing exercises – you and they are training their brain!
- Intervene early and intensively – repetition matters!
- Remember that interventions should always aim to improve activity and participation; therapy should never be mainly aimed at the improvement of impairments (Carr & Shepherd 2010).
- Always prioritise task-specific practice; however, if the patient has impairments that make it difficult to practice these tasks directly, you may also need to address

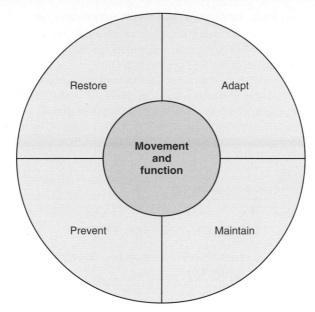

Fig. 4.3
Aims of neurological rehabilitation-RAMP.

impairments or practice specific movements either before or during a modified version of functional task practice.

- Choose exercises and activities that are meaningful for the patient.
- Consider exercise programs for independent practice.
- Consider how you can support self-efficacy (confidence) and self-management in your patients (see Jones & Kulnik 2018).
- Focus also on health promotion through lifestyle modifications and behaviour change with your patients (Dean 2009).
- Encourage fitness with a focus on health and well-being through participation in enjoyable physical activity.
- Focus also on the health and well-being of the carer to reduce caregiver burden and burnout, providing information, education and skills training (Krishnan et al 2017).

Evaluation
It is important to regularly review your treatment plan by:
- measuring outcome and progress towards goals;
- considering modification to the plan, transfer of care, or discharge; and
- planning the next review.

RECORD KEEPING: DOCUMENTING YOUR INTERVENTION

The physiotherapist should clearly document all aspects of patient management, including the results of the assessment, diagnosis, prognosis, plan of care, intervention and outcome (Standard 2.5.1 from WCPT 2011b).

A problem-oriented medical record (POMR) system is frequently used in health care. A POMR consists of baseline data, a problem list, a plan of care for each problem and progress notes (Kettenbach 2003). The POMR charting system is also known by the acronym SOAP (Box 4.6 & 4.7). Box 4.8 sums up essential record keeping rules.

Box 4.6 SOAP (Quinn & Gordon 2003)

- **Subjective**
  What the patient says about the problem/intervention.
- **Objective**
  The therapist's objective observations and treatment interventions (e.g. range of motion (ROM)).
- **Assessment**
  The therapist's analysis of the various components of the assessment.
- **Plan**
  How the treatment will be developed to reach goals.

Box 4.7 SOAP Example

- **Subjective**
  Patient reports not feeling well today 'I'm very tired'.
- **Objective**
  Strengthening exercises in standing - patient performed hip extension and abduction; 50 reps. Patient performs home exercise program (HEP) with supervision in evenings with wife.
- **Assessment**
  Patient continued with evening exercise program, which has resulted in increase in lower extremity (LE) strength. Ambulation not attempted because of patient's report of fatigue. Should be able to tolerate short distance ambulation within the next 2–3 days.
- **Plan**
  Increase strengthening ex. reps to 50 × 2 as able; attempt ambulation again 1/7.

Box 4.8 Record Keeping Rules

- Each page must contain patient identifiers.
- Write neatly and legibly with proper spelling/grammar.
- Use only blue or black ink (nonerasable).
- Use authorised abbreviations.
- Show any change in therapy parameters.
- Date/time of care and sign all notes.
- Maintain records for at least 7 years (or until a minor is 25 years of age).
- Be factual (objective).
- Errors should be crossed out and initialled.
- Store records securely.

PUTTING IT ALL TOGETHER: A CASE SCENARIO

A patient case scenario is used to illustrate how the assessment process leads to goal setting and intervention planning.

The patient assessment is outlined in Table 4.4.

The clinical reasoning form is presented in Table 4.5.

The therapist in this case has hypothesised that the loss of sitting balance/difficulty with ability to transfer/move from sitting to standing are caused by:

- weakness and loss of control in the trunk;
- loss of voluntary/selective movement in the leg – insufficient hip/knee extension and inability to depress the leg into the supporting surface;
- ankle/foot weakness and loss of ankle joint range of motion; and
- impaired lower leg proprioception.

Table 4.4 Example of an assessment of a patient poststroke

History of present complaint:	59-year-old female admitted from an acute hospital to inpatient rehabilitation unit. History of code stroke activated after falling from her bed because of left-sided weakness upon waking. Diagnosis of R middle cerebral artery infarct with left hemiplegia CT head showed large right MCA infarct. Medical plan: For Echo = Holter (Cardiac monitoring) as inpatient and Thrombophilia screen = vasculitis and commenced on Asasantin Medications: Asasantin Citalopram Perindopril Atorvastatin
Past medical history:	Nil of note

continued

Table 4.4 Example of an assessment of a patient poststroke—cont'd

Social history and environment:	<ul><li>Works × 2 days a week at local preschool</li><li>Living in her own home with her husband in a 2-storey home with 9 stairs</li><li>She has 2 grown-up children who do not live at home</li><li>Smoker × 10 a day</li><li>Hobbies – walking her dog</li><li>No history of falls before this episode</li></ul>
Previous mobility:	<ul><li>Previously independently mobile unaided with nil issues</li><li>Usually fit and active taking the dog for an hour-long walk every day</li><li>Attends local gym × 3 week</li></ul>
Expressed goals:	<ul><li>I really want to get home by the end of the week</li><li>I need to go outside somehow for a smoke</li></ul>
Cognition/ communication:	<ul><li>Alert, orientated, motivated to participate</li><li>Consent – YES</li><li>Limited insight into her functional abilities, appears to understand all information given to her</li><li>Expresses herself well</li><li>Poor concentration on task at present</li></ul>
Pain:	<ul><li>Nil at rest</li><li>Reports some pain on moving arm - 3/10 VAS</li></ul>
General observations:	<ul><li>Left lower facial paralysis</li><li>Lying asymmetrically in bed</li><li>Note lack of spontaneous movements on left</li></ul>
R upper limb:	<ul><li>Full range of movement</li><li>Muscle power 5/5</li><li>Sensation intact</li><li>Coordination NAD</li></ul>
L upper limb:	<ul><li>On palpation: no glenohumeral joint (GHJ) subluxation, head of humerus internally rotated and sitting anterior in glenoid fossa</li><li>Full passive ROM of GHJ, elbow, radio ulnar joint (RUJs), wrist and fingers</li><li>Some activity all muscle groups, not full range antigravity</li><li>Poor proximal stability when moving distally especially shoulder girdle and GHJ</li><li>In sitting, poor shoulder girdle stability whilst raising arms and reaching – shoulder hitches into elevation, shoulder flexion (60 degrees; abduction 20 degrees), elbow flexion (30 degrees). Minimal movement of wrist/fingers noted. No selective movement at wrist or fingers. All movements slow and effortful</li><li>When arms supported on table, patient able to supinate – half range, no active pronation, wrist extension with forearm support. Minimal finger flexion/extension with sensory facilitation</li><li>Tone: hypotonia throughout</li><li>Sensation light touch R = L, sensory inattention to left. Proprioception R = L</li><li>Coordination: not tested as limited activity</li></ul>

Table 4.4 Example of an assessment of a patient poststroke—cont'd

R lower limb	<ul><li>Full range of movement</li><li>Muscle power 5/5</li><li>Sensation intact</li><li>Coordination NAD</li></ul>
L lower limb	ROM, reduced external rotation left hip compared with right, hip extension appears to be limited by hip flexor muscle tightness. Note dorsiflexion −5 degrees limited by plantar flexor muscle tightness Motor control **Sitting**<ul><li>Lifts leg in flexor pattern through half range. Ankle dorsiflexion with supination noted during lift of leg. Able to extend knee 50 degrees with ankle plantarflexion. Minimal ability to isolate active knee or ankle flexor movements</li></ul>Supine<ul><li>Active hip and knee synergistic flexor and extensor movements through available range</li><li>Unable to place or maintain foot on bed in bridging position Left leg assisted to flexion by therapist, able to 'bridge', needs manual cueing to maintain level pelvis and left knee stable<ul><li>Tone: decreased compared with right</li><li>Sensation light touch R = L, sensory inattention to left. Proprioception R = L</li><li>Coordination: dysmetric</li></ul></li></ul>
Bed mobility	<ul><li>Independently rolls to L side; initiates with R arm and head</li><li>Independently moves up the bed using right leg ++</li><li>Able to bridge with assistance, uses right leg mainly and weight shift to left only</li><li>Able to roll onto R side with verbal cueing and minimal assistance for L leg, patient can activate leg muscles to assist movement to side lying</li></ul>
Lying to sitting	<ul><li>Overactive right and limited use of left UL and LL to assist</li><li>Sits up by pulling up with right arm and sitting straight up in bed. Able to perform with ×1 assist via side lying</li></ul>
Sitting on edge of bed	<ul><li>Observation: head slightly rotated and side flexed to right</li><li>Trunk side flexed to right, with elongated, low tone trunk on left, decreased postural control in sitting. Uneven weight-bearing in sitting. Left foot not fully in contact with the floor</li></ul>Sitting on bed with R arm support<ul><li>Able to initiate forward flexion/extension, needs manual and verbal cueing to maintain position</li><li>Able to reach out of base of support to right with right arm, decreased ability to return to midline. When attempting to reach to left, displaces trunk posteriorly</li></ul>

Table 4.4 Example of an assessment of a patient poststroke—cont'd

Vision	• Visual fields intact • Horizontal or vertical gaze – no saccadic eye movements • Visual inattention to left
Sit to stand	• Tending to pull up to stand, overusing right side • Assistance of 1 needed to position foot • Verbal cueing to bring trunk forward to stand. Unable to maintain weight through L foot as standing • Stands with × 2 assistance and verbal cueing. Unable to maintain knee in extension once standing; knee gives way, needs support of 1 • Arm postures in 20 degrees elbow flexion during attempt to stand, no posturing during sitting
Standing balance	• Poor LL control on left in standing • Pulling with right hand Unable to stand without support of 1–2 assist
Transfers bed to chair	Transfer to right × 2 with assistance of 1 behind to assist in weight transfer and in front to brace left knee When fatigued may require stand lifter
Gait	Unable to assess
Stairs/running	Unable to assess
Activity restrictions	Relevant impairments
1. Unable to balance and perform washing and dressing activities in sitting 2. Unable to transfer from chair/bed/plinth, independently 3. Unable to move from sitting to standing independently	1. Weakness in leg, hip, knee, foot 2. Weakness in trunk (loss of trunk–limb linked patterns) 3. Decreased hip and ankle range 4. Inability to bear weight through left leg in extension phase of stand/transfer 5. Unable to transfer weight between legs during extension phase of transfer/stand 6. Loss of trunk stability in sitting and standing

R, Right; *CT*, computed tomography; *MCA*, middle cerebral artery; *VAS*, visual analogue scale; *L*, left; *ROM*, range of movement.

Table 4.5 Clinical reasoning form for the case scenario

Problem list	Causes/sources	Therapy aim/client goal	Treatment plan
Cognition ● Decreased insight ● Concentration span of 1–2 minutes at present and easily distracted	R CVA	Early family meeting to support patient's goal re: DC Over next 2–3 weeks increase time spent focused on activity from 2 min to 20 min	Work with client, staff, carers to keep patient safe, discuss abilities/limitations Keep therapy sessions short Timetable all sessions Possible use of private spaces to assist with focus
Left UL ● Pain in left arm on movement ● GHJ sitting anterior in glenoid fossa ● Low tone and reduced activity in scapular and throughout upper limb ● Sensory inattention	Poor resting position of GHJ: decreased management strategies for UL in lying, sitting and standing		Education to patient/staff regarding positioning and use of available muscles Repositioning techniques Realign left GHJ before beginning ROM activities FES, bilateral techniques Functional strengthening – using activity that she has in a functional way, mirror therapy, motor imagery Use of gaming to facilitate activity Programme of exercise in her room – encouraging independent practice

Table 4.5 Clinical reasoning form for the case scenario—cont'd

Problem list	Causes/sources	Therapy aim/client goal	Treatment plan
Left LL ● Low muscle tone ● Some specific muscle tightness – hip, foot ● LL moving in synergies	Decreased activation muscles in left LL	Maintain ROM all joints Strengthen lower limb	Gastrocnemius/soleus/hip flexor stretches Bridging Sit to stand practice Encouraging weight-bearing out of synergistic pattern – abduction and extension of LL Progress to BWS treadmill training/robotics programme of exercises in her room for independent practice
Trunk ● Overactive right side with poor activity and elongation on left with loss of control ● Uneven weight-bearing and standing ● Poor ability to reach out of BOS and return to midline	Right side overactive to assist in keeping up against gravity Using right leg ++ standing – poor activation left LL, decreased weight-bearing and activity left trunk LL, especially inactive foot – poor acceptance of BOS	Aim to decrease right-side overactivity and increase left-side inactivity and midline awareness Sit unsupported, hands on lap 1–2 weeks	Sitting practice – use of towel to get even weight-bearing and midline awareness Pelvic tilting – anterior and lateral Reaching out of BOS Head turning and interacting with the environment Exercises from Trunk Impairment Scale to facilitate trunk activation Sit to stand with support Standing with support

Function		Goals	Treatment
Function • Overactive right side throughout functional activities • Poor activation on left, decreased awareness of midline • Needs assistance to move from lying to sitting to standing • Transfers to right × 2	Decreased activity and function on left Prolonged bed rest: deconditioning and poor initiation of functional tasks	Rolling in bed independently 1 week Lie to sit and sit to lie independently 3 weeks Sit to stand with close standby 2–3 weeks Standing with close standby for a few seconds 2–3 weeks Transfer to right and left with × 1 assist 2–3 weeks	UL and LL strengthening and balance Cardiovascular training Practice task daily facilitating normal movement Practice safe transfer techniques with nursing staff and carers as able
Low postural tone	Right CVA and prolonged bed rest		To sit out of bed after breakfast – a tabled sitting regimen Incorporate standing with support during ADL tasks as able Engage in activities on ward Encourage support and activities from family members
Visual inattention to left	Right CVA	To scan to left without external cueing 3 weeks	Practice scanning environment when sitting and supported standing and later when walking/moving around the ward
Decreased cardiovascular fitness	Prolonged bed rest	To be active achieving moderate exertion on the (BORG) perceived rate of exertion scale	UL and LL arm and leg cycle, increase repetitions of practice

Table 4.5 Clinical reasoning form for the case scenario—cont'd

Problem list	Causes/sources	Therapy aim/client goal	Treatment plan
Unable to return home at present Has 9 stairs at home that unable to negotiate	Currently not enough activity on left side to stand/walk/use stairs	To discuss situation with OT/case workers/social workers/patient/family re: use of upstairs and assess needs for day leave. To discuss with occupational therapist re: review of home situation and possible need for home modification	Involve family members/carers in discussing home options Work collaboratively with OT re: home modifications If using down stairs of home only, simulate home setup and practice with family/carers re: transfers and activities from home
Smoker × 10 a day	Premorbid addiction	Involve councillors specifically trained regarding this. Use motivational interviewing skills to help decrease or stop smoking	
Unable to work at present as primary school teacher? Financial issues	Not physically able to return to work	Discuss with patient/family and refer to social worker to delve further	
Limited family involvement in patient therapy	Time poor, lack of therapist's discussion	Family members to attend therapy sessions as able and be involved in encouraging independent practice	Family members to attend therapy sessions as able and be involved in encouraging independent practice

R, Right; CVA, cerebrovascular accident; DC, discharge; UL, upper limb; GHJ, glenohumoral joint; ROM, range of movement; FES, functional electrical stimulation; LL, lower limb; BOS, base of support; ADL, activities of daily living; OT, occupational therapist.

References

Bland, M.D., Whitson, M., Harris, H., Edmiaston, J., et al., 2015. Descriptive data analysis examining how standardized assessments are used to guide post–acute discharge recommendations for rehabilitation services after stroke. Physical Therapy 95, 710–719.

Bovend'Eerdt, T.J.H., Botell, R.E., Wade, D.T., 2009. Writing SMART rehabilitation goals and achieving goal attainment scaling: a practical guide. Clinical Rehabilitation 23, 352–361.

Carr, J., Shepherd, R., 2010. Neurological Rehabilitation: Optimizing Motor Performance. Churchill Livingstone Elsevier, New York.

Cassidy, E., Wallace, A., Bunn, L., 2018. Observation and analysis of movement (chapter 3). In: Lennon, S., Ramdharry, G., Verheyden, G. (Ed.), Physical Management for Neurological Conditions, fourth ed. Elsevier Science, London.

Chartered Society of Physiotherapy (CSP), 2014. Guidance on manual handling in physiotherapy, fourth ed. CSP, London, UK. Available at: www.csp.org.uk.

Dean, E., 2009. Foreword from the special issue editor of 'Physical therapy practice in the 21st century: a new evidence-informed paradigm and implications'. Physiotherapy Theory and Practice 25, 328–329.

Fulk, G., Field-Fote, E.C., 2011. Measures of evidence in evidence-based practice. Journal of Neurological Physical Therapy 35 (2), 55–56.

Jones, F., Kulnik, S.T., 2018. Self-management. In: Lennon, S., Ramdharry, G., Verheyden, G. (Eds.), Physical Management for Neurological Conditions, fourth ed. Elsevier Science, London.

Kettenbach, G., 2003. Writing SOAP Notes. FA Davis, Philadelphia.

Kilbride, C., Cassidy, E., 2009a. The acute patient before and during stabilisation: stroke, traumatic brain injury (TBI) and Guillain–Barré syndrome (GBS). In: Lennon, S., Stokes, M. (Eds.). Pocketbook of Neurological Physiotherapy. Elsevier Health Science, London.

Kilbride, C., Cassidy, E., 2009b. The stable acute patient with potential for recovery: stroke, TBI and GBS. In: Lennon, S., Stokes, M. (Eds.). Pocketbook of Neurological Physiotherapy. Elsevier Health Science, London.

Kimberley, T.J., Novak, I., Boyd, L., Fowler, E., 2017. Stepping up to rethink the future of rehabilitation: IV STEP considerations and inspirations. Pediatric Physical Therapy S76–S85.

Krishnan, S., York, M.K., Backus, D., Heyn, P.C., 2017. Coping with caregiver burnout when caring for a person with neurodegenerative disease: a guide for caregivers. Archives of Physical Medicine and Rehabilitation 98 (4), 805–807.

Lennon, S., 1995. Using standardised scales to document outcome in stroke rehabilitation. Physiotherapy 81 (4), 200–202.

Lennon, S., Bassile, C., 2018. Guiding principles of neurological rehabilitation. In: Lennon, S., Ramdharry, G., Verheyden, G. (Eds.), Physical Management for Neurological Conditions, fourth ed. Elsevier Science, London.

Levack, W., 2018. Goal setting in stroke rehabilitation. In: Lennon, S., Ramdharry, G., Verheyden, G. (Eds.), Physical Management for Neurological Conditions, fourth ed. Elsevier Science, London.

Levin, M.F., Kleim, J.A., Wolf, S.L., 2009. What do motor recovery and compensation mean in patients following stroke? Neurorehabilitation and Neural Repair 23, 313–319.

McLoughlin, J., 2018. Common impairments and the impact on activity. In: Lennon, S., Ramdharry, G., Verheyden, G. (Eds.), Physical Management for Neurological Conditions, fourth ed. Elsevier Science, London.

O'Rourke, M., 2007. The Australian Commission on Safety and Quality in Health Care agenda for improvement and implementation. Asia Pacific Journal of Health Management 2 (2), 21.

Playford, E.D., Siegert, R., Levack, W., Freeman, J., 2009. Areas of consensus and controversy about goal setting in rehabilitation: a conference report. Clinical Rehabilitation 23, 334–344.

Quinn, L., Gordon, J., 2003. Functional outcomes - documentation for rehabilitation. Elsevier Science, St. Louis, Missouri.

Ryerson, S., 2009. Neurological assessment: the basis of clinical decision making. In: Lennon, S., Stokes, M. (Eds.). Pocketbook of Neurological Physiotherapy. Elsevier Health Science, London.

Ryerson, S.J., Levit, K.K., 1997. Functional movement re-education: a contemporary model for stroke rehabilitation. Churchill Livingstone, New York.

Schenkman, M., Deutsch, J.E., Gill-Body, K.M., 2006. An integrated framework for decision-making in neurologic physical therapist practice. Physical Therapy 86, 1681–1702.

Shumway-Cook, A., Woollacott, M.M., 2017. Motor control: translating research into clinical practice, fourth ed. Lippincott Williams & Wilkins, Baltimore.

Sullivan, K.J., Herschberg, J., Howard, R., Fisher, B., 2004. Neurologic differential diagnosis for physical therapy. Journal of Neurological Physical Therapy 28 (4), 162–168.

Tyson, S., Burton, L., McGovern, A., 2015. The impact of an assessment toolkit on use of objective measurement tools in stroke rehabilitation. Clinical Rehabilitation 29, 926–934.

Verheyden, G., Tyson, S., 2018. Standardised measurement tools. In: Lennon, S., Ramdharry, G., Verheyden, G. (Eds.), Physical Management for Neurological Conditions, fourth ed. Elsevier Science, London.

World Confederation for Physical Therapy (WCPT), 2011a. WCPT guidelines for standards of physical therapy practice. WCPT, London, UK. Available at: www.wcpt.org.

World Confederation for Physical Therapy (WCPT), 2011b. WCPT guideline for physical therapy records: record keeping, storage, retrieval and disposal. WCPT, London, UK. Available at: www.wcpt.org.

World Health Organization, 2001. International Classification of Functioning. Disability and Health: ICF. World Health Organization.

CHAPTER 5

Clinical neurology and neurological investigations

Mark Slee

INTRODUCTION

Neurology is a clinical discipline where the patient history and examination remain central to practice. This approach has in recent decades been supported by incredible advances in neurological investigation and an ever-increasing array of effective and evidence-based treatments. This chapter will briefly outline the key steps in clinical reasoning in neurology and summarise the main investigative tools available.

THE NEUROLOGICAL HISTORY

The history is the most important element in the neurological assessment and informs the approach the neurologist will take in the examination. At the end of the history, the neurologist must have generated a number of hypotheses that are then tested in examination and investigation.

During the history, the neurologist must answer the following questions:

- **Where is the lesion or lesions?** That is, the location in the neuraxis: brain/brainstem, spinal cord, plexus or peripheral nerve, neuromuscular junction or muscle?
- **What is the likely pathological process?** Is it degenerative, inflammatory, infective, vascular, infiltrative/neoplastic, paraneoplastic, electrical/channelopathic, psychogenic/functional? One of the key elements in determining this is the time course of symptom onset and symptom evolution.
- **What is the functional impact?** What are the impairments/disabilities, and what responses or adjustments have been made by the patient and the family? What is the patient's perception of the condition? In what social and psychological context is the illness occurring?

At the conclusion of the history, the neurologist must have formed:

- a principal diagnosis;
- a list of differential diagnoses;

● an understanding of functional impact; and
● an idea of the likely outcome (prognosis).

This clinical reasoning then directs the approach to the examination and, from there, relevant investigations.

THE NEUROLOGICAL EXAMINATION

The purpose of the examination is to confirm or refute the hypotheses generated by the history. In routine clinical practice, the examination is targeted—that is, specific aspects of function are examined to enable a clinical diagnosis. Cardinal patterns of neurological diseases are sought: impairments of cognition or social conduct, gait impairment, weakness, sensory disturbance, impairments of coordination or balance, sphincteric disturbances, disorder of movement. There are many possible combinations!

A full description of the neurological examination is beyond the scope of this chapter; key steps are outlined in Table 5.1.

As an example, if weakness is present, the examination aims to reveal common patterns:

● **Is it myopathic?** This commonly appears as maximal weakness in proximal muscle groups, usually symmetrically, without sensory impairment and with present tendon reflexes (example: dermatomyositis).

Table 5.1 Key steps in the neurological examination

Observation	Begins during the history taking
	● Cognitive capacity
	● Movement
	● Gait pattern
	● Posturing (e.g. dystonic, hemiparetic)
	● Presence of a movement disorder (e.g. tremor, chorea)
Examination	Based on regions (e.g. the cranial nerves) or functions affected (e.g. gait)
	● Inspection
	Scars
	Wasting
	Fasciculation
	Unwanted movement
	● Tone: Spasticity or rigidity
	● Strength
	● Reflexes
	● Sensation
	● Coordination
	● Function

- **Is it neuropathic?** This appears as distal predominant weakness, usually symmetrical, length dependent, tendon reflexes reduced or absent, sensory impairment (example: Guillain–Barré syndrome).
- **Is it pyramidal/corticospinal?** This is a pattern of relative weakness of extensor muscle groups compared with flexor muscle groups in the upper limb and vice versa in the lower limb (example: cervical spinal cord injury).
- **Is it the neuromuscular junction?** This often appears as diffuse weakness, worse after repeated contractions (fatigable), no sensory impairment, reflexes usually spared (example: myasthenia gravis).

THE NEUROLOGIST AND THE NEUROLOGICAL PHYSIOTHERAPIST

Many gains can be made for the patient when all members of the health care team are communicating well and understand each other's role. This holds true particularly for the relationship between the neurologist and neurological physiotherapist.

The neurologist has a role primarily in medical diagnosis and therapeutics and should enlist the expertise of the neurological physiotherapist in a number of common situations (Table 5.2).

The neurological physiotherapist, by dint of their expertise and training, and often the long time they spend with patients, is in a central position to inform

Table 5.2 Examples of referral for physiotherapy

Need for rehabilitation	• Enhancing recovery from significant relapse in multiple sclerosis, stroke or episode of Guillain–Barré syndrome • During or in recovery from episodes of vestibular dysfunction
Need for functional assessment	• To determine safety for discharge or design of home (or institutional) based rehabilitation
Need for physiotherapeutic diagnosis	• Particularly where deficits in other systems (e.g. musculoskeletal) affect the primary neurological condition
Need for detailed objective muscle testing	• To monitor response to therapy such as response to intravenous immunoglobulin for patients with immune-mediated neuropathy or myasthenia gravis
Need for nondrug-based strategies	• In patients with pain syndromes or musculoskeletal disease, or management of fatigue in multiple sclerosis
Need for expert gait assessment	• For example, during pre- and post lumbar puncture for patients with suspected normal pressure hydrocephalus
Need for advice and intervention in complex neurological disease	• Where there are deficits in cognition, sensory and motor system function, such as after a large hemispheric stroke • Or maximising function in neurodegenerative disease such as Parkinson's or Alzheimer's disease

the neurologist if there is concern the patient's trajectory is not as expected. This is especially important if there is concern that:

- the patient's underlying disease is progressing unexpectedly;
- there is evidence treatment is ineffective or adverse effects of therapy are present; and/or
- nonneurological factors are affecting function, such as musculoskeletal pain, instability or muscle weakness.

The neurologist and the physiotherapist should communicate regularly regarding patient outcomes. For inpatient settings, this usually occurs as part of team meetings or in ambulatory care via written correspondence.

NEUROLOGICAL INVESTIGATIONS

Investigation should be a direct extension of the process of clinical reasoning that occurred during the history and examination. It should be driven by hypothesis and with a knowledge of the relative sensitivity and specificity of the tests in question in a given clinical scenario and the potential risks (e.g. stroke after angiography) or implications to the patient or their family (e.g. a positive genetic test). Furthermore, increasingly, investigation should be undertaken with an awareness of costs to the health system. Investigations can be used in the context of diagnosis, monitoring treatment, monitoring disease progression or development of complications.

Broadly, common investigations can be grouped based on different types of investigation such as imaging, neurophysiological tests, examination of the cerebrospinal fluid, and genetic or molecular testing (Table 5.3).

IMAGING THE NERVOUS SYSTEM
Computed Tomography

Images are created from reconstructions of many single-plane ionising (x-ray) beams. The 'slices' are usually 5 to 10 mm in width from the vertex to craniocervical junction. Thinner slices can be obtained for higher resolution of orbits, the pituitary region or in computed tomography (CT) angiography. The plane can be varied to produce images in the axial, coronal or sagittal planes.

- Different tissues (bone, cerebrospinal fluid [CSF], grey and white matter, blood) are distinguished by different electron densities.
- CT is particularly useful in the acute setting because of the rapidity of imaging, ease of access and detection of a number of serious acute pathologies such as central nervous system (CNS) haemorrhage, bony fracture, stroke, abscess or space-occupying lesions.
- CT angiography is sensitive for detection of atherosclerotic disease, dissection, vascular malformation and acute arterial and venous thrombosis.

Table 5.3 Common investigations

Imaging the nervous system (structural and functional imaging)	● **Computed tomography (CT):** CT angiography / Cerebral CT perfusion studies ● Magnetic resonance imaging (MRI): MR angiography, MR spectroscopy, MR tractography / Functional magnetic resonance imaging (fMRI), positron emission tomography (PET) ● Vascular ultrasound (US) and digital subtraction angiography (DSA) in the assessment of cerebrovascular disease
Neurophysiological investigations	● Electroencephalogram (EEG) ● Somatosensory evoked potentials (SSEP) ● Visual evoked potential (VEP) ● Brain stem/auditory evoked potentials ● Nerve conduction studies ● Electromyography (EMG)
Examination of the cerebrospinal fluid (CSF)	● Analysis of pressure and constituents
Genetic and molecular testing	● Analysis of nuclear and mitochondrial DNA for disease-causing mutations ● Assessment for pathogenical autoantibodies

● Increasingly, functional imaging with CT, such as cerebral CT perfusion studies, are used to differentiate ischaemic (but viable) cerebral tissue from infarcted (nonviable) tissue in the acute management of ischaemic stroke (Fig. 5.1).
● In the spine, CT is most commonly used in the setting of trauma.
● Disadvantages of CT include the degree of ionising radiation exposure, relatively low anatomical image resolution, lack of sensitivity for some serious pathologies (e.g. CT may be normal in acute stroke, low resolution of spinal cord disease or white matter pathologies such as multiple sclerosis) and susceptibility to artifact, such as bony artifact in the posterior fossa reducing image quality.
● After intravenous contrast administration, imaging of the cranial and cervical arteries and veins can be made, and pathologies causing breakdown of the blood–brain barrier (BBB) (e.g. cerebral tumour) can be visualised.

Magnetic Resonance Imaging (MRI, MR Angiography, Spectroscopy, Tractography, Functional MRI)

The physics of producing MRI images is beyond the scope of this text. Put simply, the MR image is produced because of the variable mobility of protons in tissues and the different 'relaxation time' (T1, T2) of protons after exposure to strong magnetic fields.

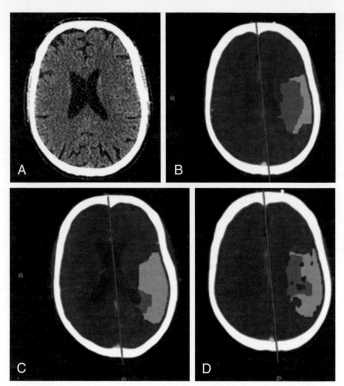

Fig. 5.1
This 75-year-old male was imaged 3 hours after the onset of acute right-sided hemiparesis, right hemianopia and global dysphasia. (A) Normal noncontrast computed tomography (CT) of the head despite major neurological deficit. (B–D) CT perfusion studies at various levels showing ischaemic but viable tissue 'penumbra' (green) and nonviable infarcted (red) tissue within the area of the left middle cerebral artery.

Differing tissues (bone, grey matter, white matter, CSF, etc.) exhibit different proton mobility and different relaxation times after exposure to strong magnetic fields, and their relative signals are altered in states of health and disease, producing differing signal intensities. MRI machines are described according to their magnetic field strength (in Tesla units, T) – most in clinical use are 1.5 T to 3.0 T, but higher-strength units are likely to become commonplace as the detail of images obtained improves substantially as field strength increases. Paramagnetic contrast agents, such as gadolinium, can be given intravenously to image pathology involving breakdown of the BBB, such as in an acute multiple sclerosis (MS) lesion or the presence of a tumour. On T1-weighted images CSF looks black, grey matter is dark grey, white matter is a lighter shade of grey, fat appears white and bone is black. On T2-weighted images, CSF is white (as is fat) and bone is dark-grey or black.

The advantages of MRI include:
- Does not involve ionising radiation.
- Very detailed images of soft tissue are obtained, including brain and spinal cord, nerve roots, ligaments and cartilage (intervertebral discs).
- Very useful for characterising white matter disease, such as in MS and ischaemic diseases such as stroke.
- Capable of imaging in many planes and very thin 'slices' (high resolution).
- Various types of MR images can be obtained that provide additional information about pathophysiology and acuity. Some common types are:
  - Diffusion-weighted imaging – very helpful in determining acute from chronic ischaemic disease (e.g. after stroke or MS relapse).
  - Susceptibility-weighted imaging, gradient-echo imaging – allow visualisation of blood and blood products.
  - FLAIR (fluid attenuation inversion recovery) imaging – suppresses the white CSF signal in cerebral ventricles to allow clearer delineation of white matter abnormality. Very useful in white matter disease such as MS.
- Can be combined with imaging of cerebral arteries and veins to produce MR angiography – very helpful in determining vessel thrombosis, stenosis, malformation or aneurysm.
- Specific brain metabolites can be imaged using MR spectroscopy – a technique very useful in determining disease states such as tumours or the presence of metabolic disease such as mitochondrial disease.
- Functional MRI (fMRI) uses MR images combined with measures of task-related cortical activation to produce images of regional cortical activity during tasks. Increasingly used in determining language localisation before surgery – for example, before epilepsy surgery.
- MR tractography – specific MR sequences that provide maps of nerve networks and tracts (e.g. pyramidal/corticospinal tracts). The images can be used to demonstrate tract integrity or disruption after trauma or head injury or to guide stimulator lead placement during procedures such as brain stimulator surgery for Parkinson's.

Some disadvantages of MRI include:
- It cannot be used with many (but not all) implanted electronic devices such as cardiac pacemakers or some metallic implants, such as certain aneurysm clips. Very careful checking is necessary.
- The MR unit 'tunnel' is usually much narrower than with CT, and some patients are unable to tolerate the enclosed space. Sedation is sometimes used.
- Often less available/accessible than CT (Fig. 5.2).

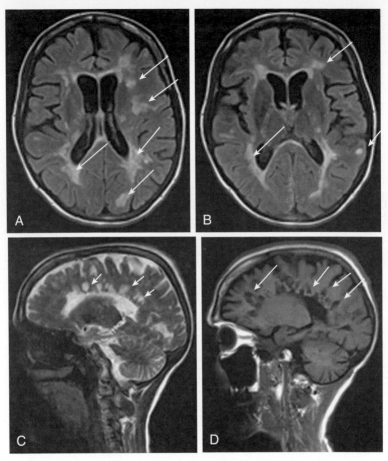

Fig. 5.2
*Various cerebral magnetic resonance imaging sequences of a patient with multiple sclerosis.
(A and B) Fluid-attenuated inversion recovery axial images demonstrating multiple regions
of focal signal hyperintensity consistent with areas of inflammatory demyelination (arrows).
(C) Midline sagittal T2-weighted image showing multiple areas of signal hyperintensity, especially in the corpus callosum (arrowheads). (D) Midline sagittal T1-weighted image showing
the similar areas as in image C but as hypointense regions indicating areas of marked axonal
loss, or 'T1-black holes' (arrows).*

Vascular Ultrasound

Colour Doppler ultrasound imaging is usually employed in the investigation of cerebrovascular disease, and in particular, where vessel thrombosis or stenosis is suspected.

- The technique is very operator dependent. It is noninvasive, largely harmless and quick to perform.
- The most common indication is investigation of anterior circulation transient ischaemic attack or stroke.
- The extracranial carotid circulation is best visualised, but images of vertebral arteries and branches of the proximal aorta are also visualised.
- Pathology such as atheromatous occlusion, stenosis or dissection can be appreciated.
- In some centres, transcranial (transtemporal) Doppler ultrasound is used to visualise intracranial vessels, monitor vasospasm after subarachnoid haemorrhage, or discover the presence of emboli.

NEUROPHYSIOLOGICAL INVESTIGATION OF NERVOUS SYSTEM FUNCTION

Electroencephalography (EEG)

EEG is a noninvasive means of measuring the electrical activity of the cerebral cortex. The signal obtained by EEG is generated by the electrical potential of cortical cells and amplified electronically to obtain the EEG record. The signal is usually measured by 21 electrodes placed on the patient's scalp. One channel, or 'line', on an EEG output represents the electrical potential difference between two recording electrodes. Electrodes are placed in frontal, temporal, parietal and occipital regions over both hemispheres.

The EEG contains waveforms of various frequencies classified into four bands: alpha (8–13 Hz), beta (more than 13 Hz), theta (4–8 Hz) and delta (0–4 Hz). The EEG is usually presented on a computer screen in association with video footage of the patient and the electrocardiograph so that visualisation of the patient occurs with simultaneous recording of cerebral and cardiac electrical activity. During the routine EEG, the patient is usually asked to rest with the eyes open and then closed, and then two manoeuvres that can enhance the presence of abnormalities are performed: hyperventilation and photic stimulation.

The EEG is most useful for investigation of the following disorders/situations:

- Where there is suspicion of seizures or epilepsy. A number of EEG waveform disturbances (such as generalised spike-wave discharges; see Fig. 5.3) are highly suggestive of epilepsy. However, a normal EEG does not exclude epilepsy.

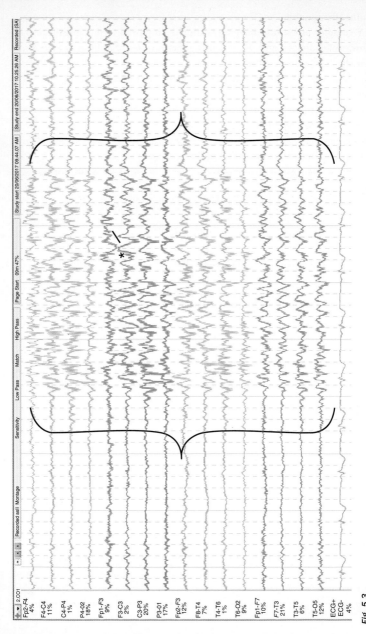

Fig. 5.3

This 10-second epoch of electroencephalography recording showing a brief (4-second) burst of asymptomatic generalised spike and wave activity (within black brackets) in an alert individual with idiopathic generalised epilepsy and history of generalised seizures. (Longitudinal bipolar montage: F-frontal, T-temporal, P-parietal, O-occipital. Even-numbered electrodes are from the right hemisphere and odd-numbered electrodes are from the left hemisphere. Example of spike [*] and wave [arrowhead] discharge in channel F3–C3).

● Disorders of consciousness or in the presence of coma. The EEG can be helpful in confirming the presence of encephalopathy and provide a guide to its severity or whether there is any focality (such as with herpes simplex encephalitis).

● Subacute or rapidly progressive dementing disorders. For example, where prion disease is suspected.

● Sleep disorders, especially where there is evidence of abnormal behaviour in sleep (parasomnias).

● In the intensive care unit where recovery of consciousness after surgery or trauma is impaired, or as part of a panel of testing of cerebral function after cardiac arrest.

Most routine EEGs take approximately 45 minutes to perform. Occasionally patients are placed in the hospital for continuous EEG and video recording.

The EEG is very prone to electrical, muscle and movement artifact, and is very dependent on the patient's level of alertness, drowsiness or sleep. Interpretation of an EEG requires significant training.

Evoked Potentials

These are surface recordings of electrical activity of sensory nerve networks whereby a sensory stimulus is applied and the conduct of potentials measured at the primary sensory cortex with scalp electrodes and also at various subcortical sensory system locations. Three main evoked potentials (EP) studies are performed: visual evoked potentials (VEP), brainstem-auditory evoked potentials (BAEP) and somatosensory evoked potentials (SSEP):

● **VEP** – One eye at a time, the patient looks at a flashing checkerboard pattern, and the subsequent electrical response at the occipital lobe is measured by a scalp surface electrode (Fig. 5.4).

  ● Is most sensitive for detecting pathology in the anterior optic pathway (optic nerve, chiasm) rather than hemispheric optic radiations.

  ● Used commonly where suspicion of MS exists because of predilection of that disease in causing inflammatory demyelinating optic nerve disease. In this situation, delay in conduction velocity is often evident.

  ● VEP abnormality can also occur in primary ocular disease.

● **BAEP** – Auditory stimulation (via headphones) causes electrical potentials that can be recorded by scalp electrodes. This tests the integrity of the entire auditory system and its brainstem connections. BAEP was commonly used to detect evidence of brainstem dysfunction before the advent of MRI because of the relative lack of sensitivity of CT imaging for posterior fossa and brainstem pathology.

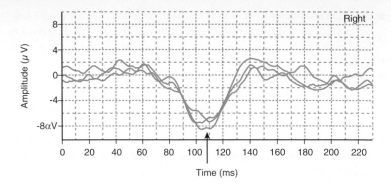

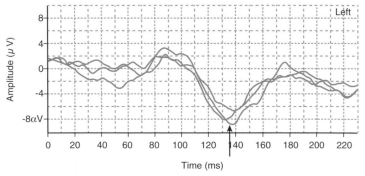

Fig. 5.4
Visual evoked potential (VEP) study in a patient with previous left optic neuritis caused by multiple sclerosis showing normal P100 response in the right eye (arrowhead at approximately 105 ms, compared with an abnormally delayed left eye P100 response at approximately 135 ms) indicating demyelinating left anterior optic pathway disease.

● **SSEP** – Electrical stimuli applied to sensory nerve fibres in the arm or leg are detected by electrodes placed over the vertebral column (to record spinal cord potentials) and over the scalp (to record cortical sensory potentials). This tests the integrity of large sensory fibres in peripheral nerves and their central connections (spinal cord and brain).

Nerve Conduction Studies and Electromyography

These allow investigation of elements of the peripheral nervous system and are a common means by which neuropathies and myopathies are investigated.

Nerve conduction studies (NCS):

- Involve the surface stimulation of motor, sensory or mixed peripheral nerves by electrical currents and recording their responses over muscle or nerve.
- Provide information predominantly from fast conducting, large myelinated fibres.
- The principal information derived from NCS relates to:
  - speed of fibre conduction;
  - size (amplitude) of response (motor or sensory); and
  - distribution of abnormality (e.g. generalised, single nerve, multifocal).
- NCS also provide information regarding probable underlying pathophysiology. For example, demyelinating peripheral neuropathies (GBS/acute inflammatory demyelinating polyneuropathy [AIDP]) are commonly associated with marked slowing of conduction speed but relative preservation of sensory and motor response amplitude. Whereas, purely axonal neuropathies are associated with no or mild conduction slowing but marked reduction in motor and sensory response amplitudes reflexing axonal loss (e.g. toxic neuropathy of chronic alcohol use).
- Common settings where NCS provide useful information are in the investigation of weakness where clinical features point to a neuropathy or myopathy as the underlying cause, or investigation of common compressive neuropathies such as carpal tunnel syndrome, wrist drop, foot drop, ulnar or common peroneal neuropathies.
- NCS also provide an objective means to monitor disease progression or response to therapy (e.g. response to treatment in GBS/AIDP) and provide prognostic information.
- Repetitive motor stimulation NCS techniques can investigate the integrity of the neuromuscular junction (e.g. investigation in myasthenia gravis).

Electromyography (EMG):

- Involves the insertion of fine needle recording electrodes across the skin, directly into muscle, from which the electrical activity of muscle is recorded at rest and during voluntary activation.
- Useful in the investigation of suspected neuropathy or myopathy and is commonly undertaken in conjunction with nerve conduction studies.
- The recording electrode samples the spontaneous and activation related motor unit potentials of surrounding muscle fibres.
- Normally innervated muscle fibres at rest are electrically 'silent'. However, denervated muscle fibres exhibit a range of abnormal discharges, such as fibrillations, and these can be detected by the recording system.

- During activation of normally innervated muscle there is orderly recruitment of motor units as the requirement for increased strength occurs. For example, in neuropathy muscle fibres are often large and polymorphic (because of reinnervation) and exhibit reduced recruitment pattern. However, in primary myopathy (such as polymyositis), the motor units are reduced in amplitude and recruitment is actually increased early as the weakened muscle seeks to activate many units early in contraction to overcome weakness.
- EMG thus can provide valuable information regarding the state of muscle health and presence or absence of denervation. It is also capable of determining distribution of denervation, which is essential in determining cause of weakness (e.g. differentiating an L5 radiculopathy from a common peroneal nerve lesion as the cause of a patient's foot drop).

OTHER INVESTIGATIONS IN NEUROLOGICAL DISEASE
Cerebrospinal Fluid (CSF) Sampling

Lumbar puncture (LP) is the means by which CSF is obtained. As the CSF is formed within the CNS, it circulates through and is absorbed within it; it can therefore provide crucial information regarding disease states. The pressure within the fluid can be measured, and the fluid can be assessed for evidence of infection, metabolic, molecular and genetic abnormalities.

- LP is usually performed by accessing the L3/L4 interspace with the patient in the lateral decubitus position and with the hips/knees gently flexed towards the abdomen.
- The CSF pressure is measured by attaching a manometer tube to the end of the LP needle and recording the height (cm) the fluid rises in the tube. Normal CSF pressure range in an adult is approximately 6 cm to 23 cm, with a wide variability recorded in the literature. Measuring pressure is useful in conditions where elevated intracranial pressure is suspected but there is no mass lesion evident on imaging, such as in idiopathic intracranial hypertension.
- Analysis of CSF fluid itself is useful in many common situations by a wide variety of techniques:
  - Suspected viral, bacterial or fungal CNS infection. These agents can be visualised directly by microscopy, can be cultured or their DNA discovered by molecular genetic techniques (polymerase chain reaction).
  - Suspected inflammatory CNS disease, such as MS, where there is intrathecal synthesis of immunoglobulin (IgG) that is not present in the systemic circulation (oligoclonal Ig bands) or infiltrating inflammatory cells directly visualised by microscopy.

- Where there may be biochemical derangement, such as elevated lactate level in mitochondrial disease or low CSF glucose in some CNS infectious diseases (e.g. tuberculosis).
- In suspected antibody-mediated CNS disease, such as neuromyelitis optica, immune-mediated encephalitis or paraneoplastic CNS disease where pathogenic autoantibodies can be detected directly in the CSF (and often also in the blood).

Muscle and Nerve Biopsy

- Direct sampling of nerve or muscle tissue (or both) is commonly undertaken and valuable in the investigation of neuromuscular disease.
- As stated earlier, NCS and EMG can provide valuable information regarding underlying pathophysiology (axonal versus demyelinating neuropathy, myopathy and the distribution of such) but may not provide specific diagnostic information. Biopsy enables direct microscopic visualisation of the tissue, analysis of cell surface markers and cellular infiltrate and evidence of infection, and provides tissue for genetic studies.

Molecular and Genetic Testing

- This field of investigation is rapidly expanding and has the potential to revolutionise clinical neurology.
- Traditionally, genetic diagnosis was limited to situations where a clinical phenotype and possibly a family history suggested a recognised monogenic disorder (e.g. adult presenting with chorea where the diagnosis of Huntington disease is suspected). The known mutation is then sought for in the individual via direct sequencing of the suspect gene via a method called *Sanger sequencing.*
- Many of the most common neurological diseases are not monogenic, but involve the complex interplay of disease-susceptibility genes and genes that confer disease protection; examples of this are MS, Alzheimer's disease and Parkinson disease.
- Disorders of mitochondrial function are often genetically determined and are diagnosed through sequencing of mitochondrial DNA; this includes disorders such as MELAS (mitochondrial encephalopathy lactic acid and stroke) and MERRF (myoclonus epilepsy and ragged red fibres).
- Many molecular and genetic tests are common practice in routine clinical neurology and enable detection of pathogens and pathogenical proteins (e.g. acetylcholine receptor antibodies in myasthenia gravis, antibodies to aquaporin-4 in neuromyelitis optica disease).

● The advent of high-throughput, commercially viable sequencing of the whole genome (genome-wide analysis) or the component of DNA that codes for proteins (whole exome sequencing) promises to revolutionise genetic diagnosis in neurology and is behind the transition of the discipline from phenotypic/phenomenological-based diagnosis towards molecular and genetic diagnosis. Key investigations are summed up in Box 5.1.

Box 5.1 Investigations and their purpose

● CT
  ● Shows brain tissues and the ventricular system, revealing haemorrhage, bony fracture, stroke, abscess or space-occupying lesions.
  ● Useful to exclude brain tumours and haemorrhage before thrombolysis.
● MRI
  ● Gives much more detailed images than CT.
  ● Useful for identifying white matter abnormalities.
● Vascular ultrasound
  ● Identifies vessel thrombosis or stenosis.
● EEG
  ● Measures electrical activity of the cortex.
  ● Useful for diagnosis of seizures or providing a guide to depth of coma.
● EP
  ● Measures electrical activity of sensory nerve networks.
  ● Useful for testing integrity of nerve networks not easily assessed by other means (e.g. optic nerves during investigation of multiple sclerosis).
● Nerve conduction
  ● Involves the surface stimulation and recording responses of peripheral nerves.
● EMG
  ● Records electrical muscle activity with a needle electrode.
  ● Differentiates between primary muscle disease and denervation of muscle.
● CSF sampling via lumbar puncture
  ● Reveals raised numbers of cells and bacteria signalling infection or detection of immune abnormalities (immunoglobulin, antibodies).
● Muscle biopsy
  ● Provides evidence of inflammation such as polymyositis or genetically determined muscle disease (e.g. muscular dystrophy).

Box 5.1 Investigations and their purpose—cont'd

- **Molecular and genetic testing**
  - Can detect genetic mutations such as in Huntington disease.
  - Can detect mitochondrial disorders and pathogenical proteins such as in myasthenia gravis.

CT, Computed tomography; *MRI*, magnetic resonance imaging; *EEG*, electroencephalography; *EP*, evoked potentials; *EMG*, electromyography; *CSF*, cerebrospinal fluid.

Further Reading

Daroff, R., et al. (Ed.), 2016. Bradley's Neurology in Clinical Practice, seventh ed. Elsevier.

Jones, R., et al. (Ed.), 2012. Netter' s Neurology, second ed. (Elsevier), Saunders.

CHAPTER 6

Management of common neurological impairments and their impact on activity

James McLoughlin

INTRODUCTION

Neurological physiotherapists need to have the knowledge and ability to identify and assess many neurological impairments, in addition to a clear understanding of how these impairments affect movement and activity. Sometimes impairments can improve with restorative rehabilitation strategies, whereas at other times these impairments will need to be monitored and managed with compensatory strategies. Prevention of secondary complications is critical. Table 6.1 lists some of the common impairments encountered in neurological practice.

Always consider the impact of impairments on activity and participation as per the International Classification of Function, Disability and Health (ICF) (World Health Organization 2001).

Impairments can be:

● Primary: directly related to neurological injury or pathology.
● Secondary: emerging from adaptations/compensations. Think how these secondary issues can be prevented!

Table 6.1 Common neurological impairments

Weakness	Upper motor neurone weakness
	Lower motor neurone weakness
Fatigue	General fatigue
	Motor fatigue
Disorders of muscle tone	Hypertonus
	Spasticity
	Hypotonus
	Involuntary muscle spasms
	Rigidity
	Dystonia

(continued)

Table 6.1 Common neurological impairments—cont'd

Disorders of coordination	Cerebellar ataxia
	Sensory ataxia
	Resting tremor
	Loss of dexterity
Disorders of motor planning	Apraxia
	Bradykinesia
	Akinesia
	Freezing of gait
Vestibular disorders	Peripheral vestibular disorders
	Central vestibular disorders
Disorders of visuospatial perception	Hemianopia
	Unilateral spatial neglect
	Contraversive pushing
Disorders of sensation	Sensory loss
	Paraesthesia/dysaesthesia
	Pain
Secondary complications	Contracture
	Physical inactivity and deconditioning
	Learned nonuse

Upper motor neurone (UMN) syndrome:

- Negative features: weakness, slowness and loss of skill.
- Positive features: increased muscle tone and hyperreflexia.
- Influenced by:
  - Velocity-dependent 'hypertonus' (increases in muscle tone)
  - Hyperreflexia, clonus and Babinski sign
  - Spasticity: increases in muscle tone and hyperreflexive responses (Stevenson 2010)
- Motor fatigue and balance impairments can influence movement adaptations.
- Coexisting impairments in motor planning, visuospatial awareness and cognition often also affect movement behaviour.

WEAKNESS

- Can be central (UMN) or peripheral (lower motor neurone [LMN]). **Table 6.2** lists some of the different features associated with UMN and LMN weakness.
- Some conditions such as motor neurone disease can result in both UMN and LMN signs.

Table 6.2 Differentiating UMN weakness from LMN weakness

UMN weakness	LMN weakness
● A lesion to descending tracts at any level above the anterior horn of the spinal cord in either the spinal cord itself, brainstem or brain.	● Lesions at the level of the anterior horn in the spinal cord or the LMN output below this level
Clinical signs: ● Initial paralysis or paresis ● Reduced skill/dexterity ● Hyperreflexia ● Hypertonus ● Weakness	Clinical signs: ● Paralysis or paresis ● Flaccidity ● Hyporeflexia ● Reduced muscle tone ● Muscle fasciculation

UMN, Upper motor neurone; *LMN*, lower motor neurone.

Aim of intervention:
● Improve muscle recruitment and control and then develop strength and endurance in key functional movements.
● Limit any decline; maintain and/or increase muscle strength where possible.

FATIGUE

Chronic fatigue is one of the most common self-reported symptoms in people with neurological disorders. Fatigue permeates all facets of life and can heavily affect employment and quality of life. Sleep, pain and depression can have a strong relationship with fatigue, as well as the side effects of many medications. Fatigue is often a major barrier to exercise and physical activity.

Kluger et al (2013) defines fatigue as 'a subjective sensation of weariness, increasing sense of effort, mismatch between effort expended and actual performance, or exhaustion'.

Fatigue also affects cognitive function, including processing speed (Barr et al 2014), which in turn affects other impairments and activities such as:
● Balance and gait (Morris et al 2016)
● Falls risk (Hoang et al 2016)
  Aim of intervention:
● Monitor motor fatigue with performance.
● Design programmes that incorporate frequent rests and consider the risk of falls and injury.

DISORDERS OF TONE

Hypertonicity, spasticity, spasms, rigidity and dystonia are all impairments that describe different aspects of increased muscular activity resulting from injury to different areas of the CNS. Sometimes these terms are used interchangeably, and they may co-occur, making clinical reasoning and treatment selection challenging. Therapists need to be aware of the exact definitions of tone-related impairments.

There are usually three main reasons for resistance to passive movement in neurological conditions (Vattanaslip et al 2000):

- Spasticity: malalignment can cause pain by adversely stressing interconnecting muscle tissue and joint structures (Thompson et al 2005).
- Thixotropy: stiffness in muscles, which is dependent on the history of the limb movement.
- Contracture: affected muscles adopt a shortened position in abnormal limb and trunk postures, which may eventually result in soft tissue shortening and biomechanical changes in the contracted muscles.

Aim of intervention:

- Disorders of tone can affect posture and movement, yet tone may not need to be directly targeted in therapy. Strength, power and neuromuscular control are the key targets for therapy intervention.

Hypertonus

Hypertonia refers to the 'stiffness' of a muscle to passive movement (Sheean & McGuire 2009). Hypertonus can be observed during both active and passive movements. It is influenced by sensory input, effort and other more global postural demands on movement (Stevenson 2010). It is critical to identify hypertonic muscles that remain in a shortened position, as this can quickly lead to contracture.

Some key interventions aimed at improving movement performance and activity, thus affecting indirectly on hypertonus, include the following:

- Altering sensory inputs and improving postural stability with either tactile hands-on input or passive assistance such as seating systems and supports can enhance the patient's ability to move (Kheder & Nair 2012).
- Task-specific practice (French et al 2016). The other advantage of task-specific practice is that it allows for greater autonomy and dose, particularly for those capable of practicing tasks outside of closely supervised therapy sessions.
- Strength training (Veerbeek et al 2014).

Why is hypertonus important?

- Hypertonic muscles that remain in a shortened position can quickly lead to contracture.
- External triggers such as painful, noxious stimuli and infection usually increase hypertonus. This can help identify hidden complications such as pressure sores or urinary tract infections.
- In some circumstances, hypertonus may provide stability.

● Care must be taken if considering reducing tone with antispasmodic medications, as this may unintentionally lead to further weakness and instability in some patients.

Spasticity (Summed up from De Baets et al (2018) with Permission)

Spasticity presents with increases in muscle tone and hyperreflexive responses (Stevenson 2010). It is characterised by disordered sensory-motor control resulting from a UMN lesion, presenting as intermittent or sustained involuntary activation of muscles (Pandyan et al 2005). Spasticity may cause additional unwanted effects such as pain, deformity and impaired function leading to activity limitations and participation restrictions for the patients, as well as everyday care issues for the caregivers (see key messages in Box 6.1).

Aim of intervention:

● To improve function, pain or risk of further deterioration (Thompson et al 2005). If spasticity is present as a symptom without other adverse effects, then intervention is not required (RCP et al 2009).

Box 6.1 Spasticity: Key messages

> ● Spasticity may be focal (localised to a specific anatomical area affecting one or two muscle groups or generalised [affecting the whole body] Royal College of Physicians [RCP] et al 2009).
> ● Spasticity will respond to focal (e.g. botulinum toxin-A; BoNT) or systemic antispasmodic medications (e.g. Baclofen).
> ● Electromyography is usually needed to differentiate between spasticity and contracture.
> ● Passive movement, active movement or positioning and interventions such as splinting or casting can achieve muscle stretch; however, current reviews have not supported these interventions for maintaining muscle length, particularly in the acute period immediately after insult (Katalinic et al 2010).
> ● In moderate to severe spasticity, pharmacological treatment may be needed to support an effective management programme (Stevenson 2010).
> ● A combination of physical and pharmacological methods within an interdisciplinary team approach are key to providing optimal spasticity control for patients and facilitating their rehabilitation or management.

Hypotonus

Hypotonus can also be observed and assessed with both passive and active movements (see Box 6.2). Many neurological populations present with hypotonus as

Box 6.2 Hypotonus: Key messages

- Patients may have difficulty in generating muscle activity because of reduced tension and 'readiness' in the muscle.
- Can result in slower movements.
- Can result in changes in joint stability and flexibility.
- Patients with hypotonic postural muscles often use more inactive, stable postures against gravity.
- Consider combining quick stretch with faster muscle activity with strength and power training during therapy.

measured by reduced resistance to passive movement. For example, hypotonus can be seen in cerebellar ataxic patients. Even early after stroke-related UMN lesions, paresis presents as 'low tone', possibly caused by changes in supplementary motor areas of the cortex, before activity-dependent adaptations lead to a hypertonic presentation (Florman et al 2013).

Dystonia

Dystonia is defined as a movement disorder characterised by sustained or intermittent muscle contractions causing abnormal, often repetitive, movements, postures or both (Albanese et al 2013). This means essentially excessive muscle activity where unwanted movements occur (see key messages in Box 6.3).

Aim of intervention:

- To improve voluntary range and control of movement, reduce tension and relieve pain (Bleton 2010) (Table 6.3).

Box 6.3 Dystonia: Key messages

- Can be present in any focal muscle group.
- Can be triggered by either postural or task-specific functional activities, or can even occur spontaneously.
- Specific muscle groups commonly affected may include cervical (spasmodic torticollis), wrist and hand (writer's cramp) and around the eyelid (blepharospasm).
- The underlying physiological cause is not well understood, but is believed to be associated with maladaptive neuroplastic changes in areas of the central nervous system (CNS) that integrate somatosensory input for movement (Stahl & Frucht 2016).
- Affects many facets of daily life, including chronic pain, balance/mobility, employment and driving.

Involuntary Muscle Spasms

Spasms may occur spontaneously or in response to the environment or the patient being moved; they are often triggered by some sensory or visceral stimuli (Nair & Marsden 2014) (see Box 6.4).

Aim of intervention:

● To explore postural control, injury management and other biomechanical influences that are commonly targeted within specific neurological physiotherapy.

Box 6.4 Spasms: Key messages

● Identify triggers such as skin lesions, pressure ulcers, musculoskeletal pains, ill-fitting splints or infections (especially urinary tract infections).
● Seating systems can be designed to minimise spasms and improve comfort and control.
● Unexpected spasms can limit standing mobility and can contribute to unexpected falls.
● Direct communication with medical colleagues is also needed to explore the medical options that may target spasms, pain and/or sleep.

Table 6.3 Interventions for dystonia

The addition of specific exercise-based physiotherapy may further improve symptoms and possibly allow for lower doses of botulinum toxin and more effective management.	Ramdharry (2006)
Exercises may focus on recruitment and strengthening of muscles that oppose the dystonic movement.	Bleton (2010)
The identification and use of somatosensory facilitation to relieve dystonic postures with 'sensory tricks' may help with self-management.	Franco and Rosales (2015)

Dyskinesias

Dyskinesias are another form of abnormal involuntary choreiform or athetoid movements. A more common dyskinesia observed within neurorehabilitation are dyskinesias associated with Parkinson's (Pilleri & Antonini 2015). Onset of dyskinesias is caused by a combination of chronic levodopa use and disease-related degenerative factors leading to postsynaptic changes to dopamine receptor sensitivity.

Rigidity

Rigidity is bidirectional; it refers to increased tone where passive movement of the peripheral joints may be difficult, even when considerable force is applied. It often occurs in people after traumatic brain injury or in people with Parkinson's.

Rigidity in Parkinson's has a lead-pipe nature of resistance that is velocity independent to the movement direction, usually tested by flexing and extending the wrist or elbow. The term *cogwheel rigidity* describes the rigidity felt in the presence of an underlying tremor. Rigidity can contribute to the overall flexed posture seen in Parkinson's and can lead to joint, tendon and muscle changes with possible associated pain.

Aim of intervention:

- Physical therapy alone is unlikely to affect rigidity, and pharmacological management (e.g. dopamine replacement) may diminish as the condition progresses. Physical therapy aims to optimise function and independence to improve quality of life, and to manage physical decline (Keus et al 2014). Physical interventions for people with Parkinson's fall broadly into three categories (Keus et al 2014):
  - exercise (related to conditioning);
  - practice (related to motor learning and performance); and
  - movement strategy training.

DISORDERS OF COORDINATION
Cerebellar Ataxia

Lesions to the cerebellum or its incoming or outgoing connections can lead to problems with the temporal and spatial control of movement (Therrien & Bastian 2015). Often seen in people with multiple sclerosis, patients with ataxia can present with:

- clumsiness;
- unsteady gait;
- impaired eye and limb movements;
- oculomotor changes such as gaze-evoked nystagmus;
- problems with articulation of speech (dysarthria); and
- tremor with active limb or postural muscle activity.

Coordination changes with cerebellar ataxia can be described as jerky, slow and inaccurate or may be observed as tremor. Clinical terms used to describe these signs include:

- dyssynergia – decomposition of multijoint movements;
- dysmetria – variable speed, path and accuracy of movement;
- dysdiadochokinesia – slow alternating rate of movement;
- tremor – kinetic, intentional or postural tremor of varying amplitude and frequency.

Aim of intervention (Table 6.4) (Freeman & Gunn 2018):

- Use restorative strategies where appropriate.
- As disability levels increase, compensatory strategies typically become the main approach.

Table 6.4 Interventions for cerebellar ataxia

Breaking movement patterns into simpler single-joint movements; using visual and verbal cues when walking can be helpful; and loading the limbs or trunk with weights to dampen the tremor all demonstrate variable success.	Marsden and Harris (2011)
The influence of postural control needs to be explored, as postural training may also reduce limb ataxia.	Stoykov et al (2005)

- Ataxia is challenging to manage, and none of the available treatments are particularly effective (Marsden & Harris 2011; Marquer et al 2014).
- Recommendations for health care professionals on the management of people with progressive ataxia have been published by Ataxia UK (2016).

Sensory Ataxia

Reduced sensation can lead to the loss of important proprioceptive awareness and feedback needed for well-coordinated movement and balance.

Aim of intervention:

- To increase additional alternative sensory feedback through vision and tactile cues to improve motor control.

Resting Tremor

Resting tremor is the most common form of tremor seen in Parkinson's that can be observed at rest or when actively holding an unchanging posture. At present, the aetiology of tremor is unknown (Hallett, 2014).

Intention Tremor

Intention tremor can involve dyssynergia and dysmetria, often with increased oscillations or tremor as the limb actively approaches the intended target. It can be familial and commonly involves involuntary intention tremor of the hands and neck/head.

All forms of tremor can have a major impact on all aspects of social and working life. Physical interventions aim to modify the proprioceptive input to allow more control with intended movements (see **Table 6.5**).

Table 6.5 Interventions for intention tremor

Innovative technology such as vibration absorbers may emerge as effective ways of reducing tremor and improving function.	Gebai et al (2016)
External weights, peripheral cooling.	Feys et al (2005)

Loss of Dexterity

Loss of dexterity can have a dramatic effect on hand function with a major impact on overall activities of daily living.

Impaired motor dexterity can arise from:

- sensory loss;
- UMN and LMN weakness;
- tremor;
- dystonia; and
- motor fatigue.

Definition of dexterity:

Reduced individualised and selective control of each digit of the hand, reduced ability in the complex shaping of the palm/fingers to manipulate objects and reduced fine motor control (Backman et al 1992).

Aim of intervention:

- Depends greatly on the capacity for active practice. Consider behaviour modification and intense practice such as constraint-induced movement therapy (CIMT) for those with adequate active movement.
- Target particular aspects of impairments such as:
  - sensorimotor training (Carey et al 2011); and
  - part-practice of a task.

DISORDERS OF MOTOR PLANNING

Apraxia

Apraxia is defined as the lack of ability to understand an action or perform an action on command or imitation (Koski et al 2002). Dyspraxia can be very frustrating for those presenting with this disorder, and can be very difficult for family and friends to fully comprehend. There is very limited evidence to guide interventional training (West et al 2008).

Aim of intervention:

- identification of the disorder;
- education;
- support; and
- use movement re-education strategies such as:
  - pantomime and imitation gesturing and compensatory strategy training (Smania et al 2000);
  - errorless learning;
  - forward or backward chaining; and
  - sensory stimulation/cueing.

Bradykinesia/Akinesia

Bradykinesia, common in PD, is described as an overall slowness of movement with a reduction in the amplitude and speed as the movement is continued.

- Can affect all movements and postures in upper limbs and hands, facial expression and speech, as well as lower limbs and gait.
- Can respond well initially to levodopa or dopamine agonist medications. Neurological therapists need to familiarize themselves with many of the physical strategies specifically used in Parkinson's in Table 6.6.

Table 6.6 Nonpharmacological interventions for bradykinesia/akinesia

Movement strategies that focus on increasing movement amplitude can help speech and mobility	Fox et al (2012)
Aerobic exercise	Petzinger et al (2013); Schenkman (2018)
Use of external auditory or visual cues	Spaulding et al (2013)
Various genres of dance	Shanahan et al (2015)

Freezing of Gait

Freezing of gait (FOG) is common in Parkinson's and occurs as brief episodes of an absence or marked reduction of the forward progression of the feet despite the intention to walk (Heremans et al 2013). FOG has an enormous impact on function and quality of life (Walton et al 2015) and can be linked to falls and cognition deficits (Peterson et al 2016).

Aim of intervention:

- Movement reeducation using external cueing strategies, education and support with mixed effectiveness (Nonnekes et al 2015; Spaulding et al 2013).

Vestibular Disorders

Vestibular disorders can be peripheral or central. This is a specialist area of practice that requires additional postgraduate training (Cohen et al 2011). See Meldrum and McConn Walsh 2018 for further reading (see key messages in Box 6.5).

Signs of vestibular dysfunction include:

- oculomotor dysfunction such as gaze evoked and/or nystagmus or reduced gaze stability caused by altered vestibular-ocular reflex;
- reduced balance and sensitivity to various types of motion; and
- vertigo.

Aim of intervention:

- Enhance early vestibular adaptation and multisensory compensation to reduce dizziness and improve balance (Hall et al 2016).

Box 6.5 Vestibular disorders: Key messages

- Careful assessment is required to differenciate both peripheral and central vestibular signs
- Often both peripheral and central vestibular signs coexist in neurological populations
- Can contribute to reduced mobility levels, increased anxiety, reduced quality of life and falls risk

VISUOSPATIAL DISORDERS

All members of the rehabilitation team need to have an understanding of cognitive and perceptual disorders to screen and address these deficits as part of their planned intervention (see Wilson (2018) for further reading). Physical therapists should seek advice from clinical neuropsychologists and occupational therapists on patient management. Three common presentations are outlined next.

Hemianopia

Homonymous hemianopia (HH) is common after stroke and results in visual field loss on the same side of both eyes. Monitoring and encouraging early compensatory head turning are important. HH can increase the risk of falls (Ramrattan et al 2001). The impact of HH on activities of daily living may be further reduced with specific visual field training (Pollock et al 2011).

Unilateral Neglect

Unilateral neglect (UN) is commonly seen in right hemisphere stroke. Patients with UN fail to respond to any stimuli from the contralateral space (often left), with characteristic ipsilesional bias of head and eye gaze. It can have a marked effect on functional recovery (Jehkonen & Laihosalo 2006) and can be difficult to manage (Kwasnica 2002).

Contraversive Pushing (Pusher Syndrome)

Contraversive pushing indicates a postural bias toward the hemiplegic side, meaning that the patient is reluctant to bear weight on the less affected side. It presents as a characteristic 'pushing' or resistance to postural correction to vertical upright. See Karnath (2007) and Perennou et al (2008) for further reading.

SENSORY DISORDERS

Sensory Loss

Sensory loss can be associated with both central and peripheral nervous system pathology. It can contribute to the following clinical problems:

- balance and mobility;

- increase in postural sway and falls risk (Cameron et al 2008); and
- skilled hand movements for both perception and action.

Aim of intervention:

- Utilise sensory reweighting to help with adaptation of balance, as well as novel ways to enhance lower limb proprioceptive feedback.
- Consider sensory training programmes (Carey et al 2011; Meyer et al 2014).
- The addition of sensory priming such as electrical stimulation or vibration can also assist with improving upper limb function (Stoykov & Madhavan 2015).

Paraesthesia and Dysaesthesia

Paraesthesia is commonly described as 'pins and needles' and 'tingling'. If these sensations become uncomfortable, they can be termed *dysaesthesia*. Physical therapists can assess areas of paraesthesia or dysaesthesia to help pinpoint areas of nerve injury, particularly in the peripheral nervous system, often arising from compression of nerves by disc bulges, osteoarthritic changes or oedema.

Pain

Pain is defined as 'an unpleasant sensory and emotional experience associated with actual or potential tissue damage (Loeser & Treede 2008). Nerve pain diagnosis can be important, as the medical management may be more effective with medications that alter CNS responsiveness such as anticonvulsant and antidepressant drugs, as opposed to strong analgesic medications, which may have limited effects. Pain management is a specialist area of practice; see Johnson & Chen (2018) for further reading.

Chronic pain can lead to:

- maladaptive brain and immune responses;
- altered movement behaviour and fear of movement leading to:
  - ongoing pain;
  - weakness;
  - inactivity; and
  - reduced independence.

Aim of intervention:

- Education, self-management and sensorimotor learning exercises to develop new strategies that aim to gain a greater repertoire of functional movement.
- Joint assessment with experienced musculoskeletal colleagues can be helpful.

SECONDARY COMPLICATIONS

Physical therapy management should focus as much as possible on prevention of secondary complications. Three common secondary complications to consider are contracture (Box 6.6), physical inactivity and deconditioning (Box 6.7) and learned nonuse (Box 6.8).

Box 6.6 Contracture: Key messages

- Contractures can develop rapidly, so education about positioning to the patient, family, carers and the entire multidisciplinary team is critical.
- Key structural changes within the muscle are loss of sarcomeres and muscle atrophy.
- Muscles left in a shortened position can quickly lead to more permanent muscle shortening. Often this occurs with hypertonus and spasticity.
- Can lead to musculoskeletal deformity, reduced function, joint capsule and ligament changes, pain and pressure areas (Farmer & James 2001).
- Occurs commonly in at-risk groups:
  - ankle plantarflexors;
  - hip flexors;
  - shoulder internal rotators;
  - subscapularis/pectoralis minor; and
  - wrist and finger flexors.
- Interventions aim to improve range of motion and function or to assist with hygiene and/or pain and include:
  - careful positioning with preventative splinting;
  - serial casting and some orthopaedic surgical procedures may assist with gaining some increased range (Pidgeon et al 2015);
  - limited effect of prolonged stretching (Harvey et al 2017);
  - combine botulinum toxin with active rehabilitation;
  - strengthen antagonistic muscle groups through range with/without electrical stimulation; and
  - eccentric training of agonist muscles.

Box 6.7 Physical inactivity and deconditioning: Key messages

- People living with neurological conditions are faced with many barriers that make it difficult to remain physically active.
- It leads to an increase in risk of lifestyle disease such as heart disease, diabetes and forms of cancer (Mulligan et al 2012).
- Interventions need to focus on:
  - strength and cardiovascular fitness;
  - behaviour modification strategies;
  - addressing barriers to physical activity; and
  - using rehabilitation technologies such as virtual reality, robotics, exergaming and telerehabilitation, especially in the community setting.

Box 6.8 Learned nonuse: Key messages

- Learned nonuse of the hemiparetic extremity refers to compensatory movement behaviours that favour use of the less affected limb.
- Forced use of this limb can improve function using different forms of CIMT (Corbetta et al 2015).
- Principles of CIMT include (Taub et al 2013):
  - Constraint of the less affected arm/hand for 90% of waking hours;
  - Repetitive task-specific practice or practicing graded segments of tasks (shaping) from 3 up to 6 hours, and
  - Transfer package of repeated behavioural reflection to enhance real-world use of the extremity.

This chapter is an abridged version adapted from McLoughlin (2018) with permission.

References

Albanese, A., Bhatia, K., Bressman, S.B., et al., 2013. Phenomenology and classification of dystonia: a consensus update. Movement Disorders 28 (7), 863–873.

Ataxia, U.K., 2016. Management of the ataxias: towards best clinical practice, third ed. Ataxia UK, London.

Backman, C., Gibson, S.C.D., Parsons, J., 1992. Assessment of hand function: the relationship between pegboard dexterity and applied dexterity. Canadian Journal of Occupational Therapy 59 (4), 208–213.

Barr, C., McLoughlin, J., Lord, S.R., Crotty, M., Sturnieks, D.L., 2014. Walking for six minutes increases both simple reaction time and stepping reaction time in moderately disabled people with Multiple Sclerosis. Multiple Sclerosis and Related Disorders 3 (4), 457–462.

Bleton, J.-P., 2010. Physiotherapy of focal dystonia: a physiotherapist's personal experience. European Journal of Neurology 17 (Suppl. 1), 107–112.

Cameron, M.H., Horak, F.B., Herndon, R.R., Bourdette, D., 2008. Imbalance in multiple sclerosis: a result of slowed spinal somatosensory conduction. Somatosensory & Motor Research 25, 113–122.

Carey, L., Macdonell, R., Matyas, T.A., 2011. SENSe: study of the effectiveness of neurorehabilitation on sensation a randomized controlled trial. Neurorehabilitation and Neural Repair 25 (4), 304–313.

Cohen, H.S., Gottshall, K.R., Graziano, M., et al., 2011. International guidelines for education in vestibular rehabilitation therapy. Journal of Vestibular Research 21 (5), 243–250.

Corbetta, D., Sirtori, V., Castellini, G., Moja, L., Gatti, R., 2015. Constraint-induced movement therapy for upper extremities in people with stroke. Available at: http://online library.wiley.com/doi/10.1002/14651858.CD004433.pub3/pdf.

De Baets, L., Ashford, S., Devos, H., Akinwuntan, A.E., 2018. Complex case management. In: Lennon, S., Ramdharry, G., Verheyden, G. (Eds.), Physical Management for Neurological Conditions. Elsevier Science, London.

Farmer, S.E., James, M., 2001. Contractures in orthopaedic and neurological conditions: a review of causes and treatment. Disability and Rehabilitation 23 (13), 549–558.

Feys, P., Helsen, W., Liu, X., et al., 2005. Effects of peripheral cooling on intention tremor in multiple sclerosis. Journal of Neurology, Neurosurgery, and Psychiatry 76, 373–379.

Florman, J.E., Duffau, H., Rughani, A.I., 2013. Lower motor neuron findings after upper motor neuron injury: insights from postoperative supplementary motor area syndrome. Frontiers in Human Neuroscience 7, 85–110.

Fox, C., Ebersbach, G., Ramig, L., Sapir, S. 2012. LSVT LOUD and LSVT BIG: behavioral treatment programs for speech and body movement in parkinson disease. Parkinson's Disease 391946.

Franco, J.H., Rosales, R.L., 2015. Neurorehabilitation in dystonia. In: Kanovsky, P., Bhatia, K.P., Rosales, R.L. (Eds.), Dystonia and Dystonic Syndromes. Springer Verlag, Vienna. (pp. 209–226).

Freeman, J., Gunn, H., 2018. Multiple sclerosis. In: Lennon, S., Ramdharry, G., Verheyden, G. (Eds.), Physical Management for Neurological Conditions. Elsevier Science, London.

French, B., Thomas, L.H., Coupe, J., McMahon, N.E., Connell, L., Harrison, J., Sutton, C.J., Tishkovskaya, S., Watkins, C.L., 2016. Repetitive task training for improving functional ability after stroke. Cochrane Database of Systematic Reviews (11), CD006073.

Gebai, S., Hammoud, M., Hallal, A., Shaer, A.A., Khachfe, H., 2016. Biomechanical treatment for rest tremor of Parkinson's patient. In: 2016 IEEE International Multidisciplinary Conference on Engineering Technology (IMCET). https://doi.org/10.1109/IMCET.2016.7777422.

Hall, C.D., Herdman, S.J., Whitney, S.L., et al., 2016. Vestibular rehabilitation for peripheral vestibular hypofunction: an evidence-based clinical practice guideline: from the american physical therapy association neurology section. Journal of Neurologic Physical Therapy 40 (2), 124–155.

Hallett, M., 2014. Tremor: pathophysiology. Parkinsonism & Related Disorders 20 (Suppl. 1), S118–S122.

Harvey, L.A., Katalinic, O.M., Herbert, R.D., et al., 2017. Stretch for the treatment and prevention of contracture: an abridged republication of a Cochrane Systematic Review. Journal of Physiotherapy 63 (2), 67–75.

Heremans, E., Nieuwboer, A., Vercruysse, S., 2013. Freezing of gait in Parkinson's disease: where are we now? Current Neurology and Neuroscience reports 13 (6), 350.

Hoang, P.D., Baysan, M., Gunn, H., et al., 2016. Fall risk in people with MS: A Physiological Profile Assessment study. Multiple Sclerosis Journal – Experimental, Translational and Clinical 2, 2055217316641130. https://doi.org/10.1177/2055217316641130.

Jehkonen, M., Laihosalo, M., 2006. Impact of neglect on functional outcome after stroke–a review of methodological issues and recent research findings. Restorative Neurology and Neuroscience 24 (4–6), 209–215.

Johnson, M.I., Chen, C.C., 2018. Pain management. In: Lennon, S., Ramdharry, G., Verheyden, G. (Eds.), Physical Management for Neurological Conditions. Elsevier Science, London.

Karnath, H.O., 2007. Pusher syndrome—a frequent but little-known disturbance of body orientation perception. Journal of Neurology 254 (4), 415–424.

Katalinic, O.M., Harvey, L.A., Herbert, R.D., Moseley, A.M., Lannin, N.A., Schurr, K., 2010. Stretch for the treatment and prevention of contractures. Cochrane Database of Systematic Reviews (9), 1–29.

Keus, S.H.J., Munneke, M., Graziano, M., et al., 2014. European Physiotherapy Guideline for Parkinson's disease. KNGF/ ParkinsonNet, The Netherlands.

Kheder, A., Nair, K.P.S., 2012. Spasticity: pathophysiology, evaluation and management. Practical Neurology 12 (5), 289–298.

Kluger, B.M., Krupp, L.B., Enoka, R.M., 2013. Fatigue and fatigability in neurologic illnesses: proposal for a unified taxonomy. Neurology 80 (4), 409–416.

Koski, L., Iacoboni, M., Mazziotta, J.C., 2002. Deconstructing apraxia: understanding disorders of intentional movement after stroke. Current Opinion in Neurology 15 (1), 71–77.

Kwasnica, C.M., 2002. Unilateral neglect syndrome after stroke: theories and management issues. Critical Reviews in Physical and Rehabilitation Medicine 14 (1).

Loeser, J.D., Treede, R.-D., 2008. The Kyoto protocol of IASP Basic Pain Terminology. Pain 137 (3), 473–477.

Marsden, J., Harris, C., 2011. Cerebellar ataxia: pathophysiology and rehabilitation. Clin Rehabil 25, 195–216.

Marquer, A., Barbieri, G., Perennou, D., 2014. The assessment and treatment of postural disorders in cerebellar ataxia: a systematic review. Annals of Physical and Rehabilitation Medicine 57 (2), 67–78.

McLoughlin, J.V., 2018. Common impairments and the impact on activity (chapter 2). In: Lennon, S., Ramdharry, G., Verheyden, G. (Eds.), 2018 Physical Management for Neurological Conditions. Elsevier Science, London.

Meldrum, D., McConn Walsh, R., 2018. Vestibular rehabilitation (Chapter 21). In: Lennon, S., Ramdharry, G., Verheyden, G. (Eds.), Physical Management for Neurological Conditions. Elsevier Science, London.

Meyer, S., Karttunen, A.H., Thijs, V., Feys, H., Verheyden, G., 2014. How do somatosensory deficits in the arm and hand relate to upper limb impairment, activity, and participation problems after stroke? A systematic review. Physical Therapy 94 (9), 1220–1231.

Morris, R., Lord, S., Bunce, J., Burn, D., Rochester, L., 2016. Gait and cognition: mapping the global and discrete relationships in ageing and neurodegenerative disease. Neuroscience and Biobehavioral Reviews 64, 326–345.

Mulligan, H.F., Hale, L.A., Whitehead, L., Baxter, G.D., 2012. Barriers to physical activity for people with long-term neurological conditions: a review study. Adapted Physical Activity Quarterly 29 (3), 243–265.

Nair, K.P.S., Marsden, J., 2014. The management of spasticity in adults. British Medical Journal 349, 4737.

Nonnekes, J., Snijders, A.H., Nutt, J.G., et al., 2015. Freezing of gait: a practical approach to management. Lancet Neurology 14 (7), 768–778.

Pandyan, A.D., Gregoric, M., Barnes, M.P., Wood, D., van Wijck, F., Burridge, J., Johnson, G.R., 2005. Spasticity: clinical perceptions, neurological realities and meaningful measurement. Disability and Rehabilitation 27, 2–6.

Perennou, D.A., Mazibrada, G., Chauvineau, V., et al., 2008. Lateropulsion, pushing and verticality perception in hemisphere stroke: a causal relationship? Brain 131, 2401–2413.

Peterson, D.S., King, L.A., Cohen, R.G., Horak, F.B., 2016. Cognitive contributions to freezing of gait in Parkinson disease: implications for physical rehabilitation. Physical Therapy 96 (5), 659–670.

Petzinger, G.M., Fisher, B.E., McEwen, S., et al., 2013. Exercise-enhanced neuroplasticity targeting motor and cognitive circuitry in Parkinson's disease. Lancet Neurology 12 (7), 716–726.

Pidgeon, T.S., Ramirez, J.M., Schiller, J.R., 2015. Orthopaedic management of Spasticity. Rhode Island Medical Journal 98 (12), 26–31.

Pilleri, M., Antonini, A., 2015. Therapeutic strategies to prevent and manage dyskinesias in Parkinson's disease. Expert Opinion on Drug Safety 14 (2), 281–294.

Pollock, A., Hazelton, C., Henderson, C.A., et al., 2011. Interventions for disorders of eye movement in patients with stroke. Cochrane Database of Systematic Reviews (10), CD008389.

Ramdharry, G., 2006. Physiotherapy cuts the dose of botulinum toxin. Physiotherapy Research International 11 (2), 117–122.

Ramrattan, R.S., Wolfs, R.C., Panda-Jonas, S., et al., 2001. Prevalence and causes of visual field loss in the elderly and associations with impairment in daily functioning: the Rotterdam Study. Archives of Ophthalmology 119 (12), 1788–1794.

Royal College of Physicians, British Society of Rehabilitation Medicine, Chartered Society of Physiotherapy & Association of Chartered Physiotherapists Interested in Neurology, 2009. Spasticity in Adults: Management Using Botulinum Toxin - National Guidelines. Royal College of Physicians, Clinical Effectiveness and Evaluation Unit, London.

Schenkman, M., Moore, C.G., Kohrt, W.M., Hall, D.A., Delitto, A., Comella, C.L., Melanson, E.L. 2018. Effect of high-intensity treadmill exercise on motor symptoms in patients with de novo parkinson disease: a phase 2 randomized clinical trial. JAMA neurology, 75 (2), 219–226.

Shanahan, J., Morris, M.E., Bhriain, O.N., Saunders, J., 2015. Dance for people with Parkinson disease: what is the evidence telling us? Archives of Physical Medicine and Rehabilitation 96 (1), 141–153.

Sheean, G., McGuire, J.R., 2009. Spastic hypertonia and movement disorders: pathophysiology, clinical presentation, and quantification. Physical Medicine & Rehabilitation 1, 827–833.

Smania, N., Girardi, F., Domenicali, C., Lora, E., Aglioti, S., 2000/4. The rehabilitation of limb apraxia: a study in left-brain–damaged patients. Archives of Physical Medicine and Rehabilitation 81 (4), 379–388.

Spaulding, S.J., Barber, B., Colby, M., et al., 2013. Cueing and gait improvement among people with Parkinson's disease: a meta-analysis. Archives of Physical Medicine and Rehabilitation 94 (3), 562–570.

Stahl, C.M., Frucht, S.J., 2016. Focal task specific dystonia: a review and update. Journal of Neurology 264, 1536–1541.

Stevenson, V.L., 2010. Rehabilitation in practice: spasticity management. Clinical Rehabilitation 24 (4), 293–304.

Stoykov, M.E., Madhavan, S., 2015. Motor priming in neurorehabilitation. Journal of Neurologic Physical Therapy 39 (1), 33–42.

Stoykov, M.E.P., Stojakovich, M., Stevens, J.A., 2005. Beneficial effects of postural intervention on prehensile action for an individual with ataxia resulting from brainstem stroke. NeuroRehabilitation 20 (2), 85–89.

Taub, E., Uswatte, G., Mark, V.W., 2013. Method for enhancing real-world use of a more affected arm in chronic stroke: transfer package of constraint-induced movement therapy. Stroke 44 (5), 1383–1388.

Therrien, A.S., Bastian, A.J., 2015. Cerebellar damage impairs internal predictions for sensory and motor function. Current Opinion in Neurobiology 33, 127–133.

Thompson, A., Jarrett, L., Lockley, L., Marsden, J., Stevenson, V.L., 2005. Clinical management of spasticity. Journal of Neurology, Neurosurgery and Psychiatry 76, 459–463.

Vattanaslip, W., Ada, L., Crosbie, J., 2000. Contribution of thixotropy, spasticity and contracture to ankle stiffness after stroke. Journal of Neurology Neurosurgery and Psychiatry 69, 34–39.

Veerbeek, J.M., Van Wegen, E., Van Peppen, R., Van der Wees, P.J., Hendriks, E., Rietberg, M., Kwakkel, G., 2014. What is the evidence for physical therapy poststroke? A systematic review and meta-analysis. PLoS One 9 (2), e87987.

Walton, C.C., Shine, J.M., Hall, J.M., et al., 2015. The major impact of freezing of gait on quality of life in Parkinson's disease. Journal of Neurology 262 (1), 108–115.

West, C., Bowen, A., Hesketh, A., Vail, A., 2008. Interventions for motor apraxia following stroke. The Cochrane Database of Systematic Reviews 23 (1), CD004132. https://doi.org/10.11002/ 14651858.CD004132.pub2.

World Health Organization, 2001. International Classification of Functioning, Disability and Health (ICF). World Health Organization, Geneva. Available online at: http:/www.who.int/ classification/icf.

Wilson, C.F., 2018. Clinical neuropsychology in rehabilitation. In: Lennon, S., Ramdharry, G., Verheyden, G. (Eds.), Physical Management for Neurological Conditions. Elsevier Science, London.

CHAPTER 7

Respiratory management

Adrian Capp and Louise Platt

INTRODUCTION

An acute neurological insult or neurological disease may affect breathing through injury to the respiratory control centres (RCCs) or to one or more of the respiratory system sensors leading to altered rate, depth and pattern of breathing. Associated muscle weakness and fatigue will further contribute to respiratory compromise and dysfunction. Initially, this will result in dysfunction of gas exchange which can, if left uncorrected, lead to respiratory failure. If swallowing, cough and airway clearance are affected, then airway protection will be compromised resulting in possible aspiration and leading to further dysfunction of gas exchange. Changes in blood gas chemistry can lead to changes within the cerebral vasculature, which can lead to brain hypoxia and secondary brain injury. Neurological patients can also develop respiratory infections through immobility. It is therefore vital that a full respiratory assessment is completed and close liaison with the medical team and other members of the multiprofessional team (e.g. medical team, nursing team, speech and language therapy colleagues) is sought (see common problems in Box 7.1).

Box 7.1 Common problems in neurological conditions affecting respiration

- Injury to brainstem (RCCs)
- Respiratory muscle weakness
- Fatigue
- Impaired swallowing (aspiration)
- Impaired ability to cough (sputum retention/infection)
- Hypoxia

Central Nervous Control of Breathing

Breathing is coordinated through a number of cortical areas primarily located within the medulla oblongata (inspiratory and expiratory centres) and the pons (pneumotaxic and apneustic centres).

Relationship Between Brain Function and Lung Function

The relationship between brain function and lung function is critical, as the brain requires adequate oxygenation to function, and the respiratory system relies on drive from the brain to control ventilation. In neurological conditions, cerebral blood flow can be altered by:

● oedema;
● a change in blood pressure (BP);
● direct injury.

Because neurological deterioration can occur quickly, careful monitoring is essential during the acute phase. Patients with neurological conditions may be ventilated, sedated, paralysed, intubated, and admitted to intensive care during the acute phase. This may be done initially to minimise agitation arising from the negative cascade of effects of agitation leading to raised BP, raised intracranial pressure (ICP) and reduced brain oxygenation. The management aim in the acute phase is to ensure adequate oxygenation is maintained to the brain and vital organs to avoid secondary ischaemic changes; therefore treatment aims should be directed at:

● preventing sputum retention;
● optimising lung volume;
● maintaining a patent airway;
● ensuring adequate ventilation;
● preserving the integrity of the musculoskeletal system.

RESPIRATORY ASSESSMENT OF THE NEUROLOGICAL PATIENT

In conjunction with a full respiratory assessment (Bruton 2011; see key elements in Box 7.2, and red flags in Box 7.3), particular attention should be given to:

● lung function;
● peak cough flow;
● arterial blood gases;
● chest radiographs;
● respiratory patterns;
● respiratory reserve considerations for early mobilisation.

Box 7.2 Elements of a respiratory assessment (with permission from Bruton 2011)

General End-of-Bed Observations

Breathing pattern, cyanosis, distress, accessory muscle use, swallowing, speech pattern, posture

History (from Patient/Relatives/Friends)

Past medical history, history of present complaint, recent symptoms (cough/sputum/chest tightness/breathlessness), smoking history, environmental exposures (pollution/occupational), family health history, travel history, social history, drug history

Clinical Examination

Inspection – hands (finger clubbing, tremor, temperature); chest shape; breathing rate, depth, frequency, symmetry (left:right) and regularity; sputum (quantity, colour, smell); cough competence

Palpation checking for – tracheal centrality; chest pulsations/tenderness/depressions/bulges/movements/scars; tactile/vocal fremitus

Percussion – to detect chest resonance/dullness

Auscultation – to listen for presence/absence of normal or added lung sounds

Current General Status

Body temperature, blood pressure, pulse rate, fluid balance, blood chemistry, intracranial pressure

Respiratory Bedside/Laboratory Testing

Chest x-rays/other imaging, sputum culture, arterial blood gases, pulse oximetry, lung function tests (e.g. vital capacity), peak cough flow, inspiratory/expiratory pressures (mouth/sniff/transdiaphragmatic).

Box 7.3 Respiratory 'red flags' (Bruton 2011)

- General (e.g. chest pain/haemoptysis) – always needs further investigation because of potential to indicate serious pathology.
- Breathlessness or inability to talk in complete sentences at rest – breathlessness may be of sudden onset or gradual. If related to muscle weakness, it may initially be more apparent at night when lying down or sleeping.
- Accessory muscle use while at rest – normal breathing requires minimal effort, so use of additional muscles (e.g. sternocleidomastoid) indicates respiratory distress.
- Weak cough or inability to clear secretions – suggests weakness of expiratory muscles.
- Cyanosis (dusky or bluish tinge to skin) – seen around lips/tongue = central cyanosis. Usually only occurs once arterial oxygen tension falls below 8 kPa (60 mmHg) and oxygen saturation below 90%. Can be difficult to detect reliably in artificial lighting.
- Altered mental status – agitation/drowsiness. Acute confusion with breathlessness may indicate severe hypoxaemia (or sepsis/metabolic disturbance).
- Exhaustion and shallow breathing – may follow a period of 'distressed' breathing, when work of breathing overwhelms the patient and fatigue leads to ventilatory failure.
- Altered arterial blood gases – hypoxaemia with hypercapnia indicates ventilatory failure.
- Vital capacity falling below 15 mL/kg body weight indicates respiratory muscle weakness requiring ventilator support (Polkey et al 1999).

Lung Function

Inspiratory muscle weakness leads to a reduction in vital capacity (VC). VC is the volume change at the mouth between full inspiration and complete expiration (Fig. 7.1). A normal VC in the supine position indicates that respiratory muscle weakness is unlikely; however, in many neurological conditions, weakness can fluctuate; therefore the VC and oxygen saturation should be checked at regular intervals (Bruton 2011). Monitoring of VC is essential in progressive conditions such as Guillain–Barré syndrome to indicate when ventilatory support is required (see critical values in Box 7.4).

Box 7.4 Critical values of VC

- Normal values are calculated from the patient's age, height and gender.
- A fall in vital capacity (VC) by >25% in the supine position indicates significant diaphragm weakness.
- When VC falls below 1.5 L, careful monitoring is required.
- When VC falls below 1 L, ventilation may be required (Hughes & Binaries 1993).
- A patient with a VC of less than 50% of predicted value may be at risk of nocturnal hypoventilation and may benefit from further investigation and instigation of noninvasive ventilation.

Peak Cough Flow

Insufficient cough strength has a significant impact on effective sputum clearance for patients with neuromuscular weakness. Patients may have difficulty with sputum clearance as a result of inspiratory or expiratory muscle weakness or impaired bulbar function. Peak cough flow (PCF) is a measure of maximal airflow during a cough; it is a useful indicator of cough strength and effectiveness. It is important to ascertain the specific component of the cough that a patient is having difficulty with (see critical values in Box 7.5). If both inspiratory and expiratory weakness have been ruled out, then referral to a speech and language therapist should be considered for the joint assessment of bulbar function (Simonds 2016). It should be remembered that an ineffective cough may be a result of a combination of issues.

Box 7.5 Critical values of PCF (BTS Guideline, 2009)

- 360–840 L/min is normal
- <270 L/min at risk of serious infection; therefore teach airway clearance strategies
- <160 L/min may require ventilation

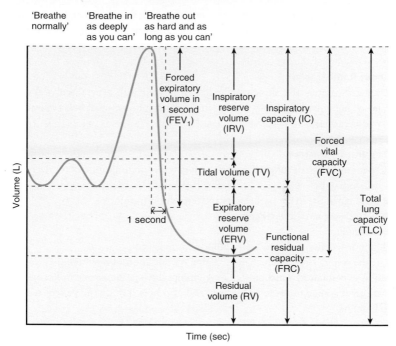

'Breathe normally'   'Breathe in as deeply as you can'   'Breathe out as hard and as long as you can'

Fig. 7.1

Lung volumes and capacities in neurological disease. From Al-Ashkar F1, Mehra R, Mazzone PJ. Interpreting pulmonary function tests: Recognize the pattern, and the diagnosis will follow. Cleveland Clinic Journal of Medicine. 2003 October;70(10):866-881. Reprinted with permission.

Arterial Blood Gases

Arterial blood gas measurement is essential; both PaO_2 and $PaCO_2$ can be affected by respiratory muscle weakness. Pulse oximetry is useful, providing a noninvasive measure of oxygen saturation (SpO_2). It can help identify problems such as atelectasis and pneumonia (see critical values in Box 7.6).

Box 7.6 Critical blood gas values (BTS 2017)

- A normal value for PaO_2 : 75–100 mmHg (10–13.3 kPa)
  - <60 mmHg < 8 kPa indicates hypoxaemia
- A normal value for $PaCO_2$: 34–46 mmHg (4.6–6.1 kPa)
  - > 45 mmHg > 6.1 kPa indicates hypercapnia
- A normal value for SpO_2: 95%–98%
  - <95% requires careful monitoring
  - <90% indicates hypoxia

Hypercapnia (increased levels of carbon dioxide) and associated acidosis (increased acidity) will often develop in the presence of significant respiratory muscle weakness with associated hypoventilation (Main & Denehy 2016).

Chest Radiographs

Chest radiographs will show volume loss associated with generalised weakness. A raised hemidiaphragm may indicate unilateral diaphragm weakness (Howard & Davidson 2003).

Respiratory Pattern

Respiratory pattern is subjective; however, it may give an indication of the degree of respiratory muscle weakness. Respiratory pattern can be affected by:

- damage to the RCCs in the pons and upper midbrain;
- respiratory muscle weakness;
- fatigue;
- abnormal alterations in arterial blood gas tensions.

If the respiratory pattern changes during mobilisation, it may indicate deterioration in respiratory function (Stiller & Phillips 2003). The degree in fluctuation from the baseline needs to be assessed and also how quickly the patient returns to baseline.

Respiratory Reserve (PaO_2/FiO_2 Ratio)

The partial pressure of oxygen (PaO_2) in arterial blood falls steadily with age, reaching approximately 10.3 kPa by the age of 60 years (West 2012). The fraction of inspired oxygen (FiO_2) can assist in the assessment of suitability for rehabilitation. This should be taken into account in conjunction with PaO_2 and reflects the respiratory reserve (Fig. 7.2; see critical values in Box 7.7).

Box 7.7 Critical values of the PaO_2/FiO_2 ratio

> - Above 300 indicates that a patient is likely to have sufficient respiratory reserve to tolerate rehabilitation.
> - Between 200 and 300 indicates marginal respiratory reserve.
> - Below 200 indicates low respiratory reserve.

The ratio between PaO_2/FiO_2 can be calculated easily and used to give an indication of a patient's ability to tolerate rehabilitation (Stiller & Phillips 2003). The use of respiratory reserve should be used in conjunction with all available parameters to assess suitability for early rehabilitation.

$$\frac{\text{Partial pressure of arterial oxygen kPa (PaO}_2)}{\text{Fraction of inspired oxygen (FiO}_2)} \times 7.5 = \text{Respiratory reserve}$$

Examples

Normal breathing room air

$$\frac{13.3 \text{ kPa}}{0.21} \times 7.5 = 475 \text{ High respiratory reserve}$$

Head injury with tracheostomy

$$\frac{10.2 \text{ kPa}}{0.30} \times 7.5 = 255 \text{ Marginal respiratory reserve}$$

Fig. 7.2
Calculation for respiratory reserve (Stiller & Phillips 2003). Examples are shown for a healthy person breathing room air and a head-injured patient.

Oxygen uptake needs to be considered, as there will be increased oxygen consumption caused by increased muscle activities such as turning and mobilising. Oxygen consumption and metabolic demands will be affected by sepsis, temperature and BP. Liaison with the dietician is important to ensure appropriate nutrition is provided to meet any changes in metabolic demands to ensure effective oxygen uptake.

Early Mobilisation
Early mobilisation in critical care has been shown to be both safe and feasible (Adler & Malone 2012, Hodgson et al 2014). The therapist must assess if there is sufficient respiratory and cardiovascular reserve before mobilising a patient. There are limited published clinical data concerning resting heart rate (HR) and BP. Key cardiorespiratory parameters that should be considered are:
● variations in BP less than 20% of baseline;
● resting HR less than 50% age-predicted maximal heart rate (Stiller & Phillips 2003).

The National Hospital for Neurology & Neurosurgery (NHNN) Local Guidelines have devised an early rehabilitation algorithm (see selected key criteria from Capp & Platt (2018); see Box 7.8 & 7.9). The decision to mobilise a patient in critical care is a multidisciplinary team decision. It is important to ensure that oxygenation is maximised to avoid or limit ischaemia. Patients must be monitored for signs of fatigue or deterioration during early mobilisation. This may indicate that the intervention is not being tolerated and needs to be adapted.

Box 7.8 Key criteria for early rehabilitation and mobilisation

- Is there sufficient cardiovascular reserve?
- Is there sufficient respiratory reserve?
- Are there patient-specific neurological considerations such as spinal precautions, vasospasm, etc.?
- Are other factors favourable such as?
  - weight;
  - safe environment;
  - appropriate staffing and expertise;
  - appropriate equipment.

Adapted from Early Rehabilitation/Mobilisation in a Neurosurgical Critical Care Unit Algorithm. The National Hospital for Neurology & Neurosurgery (NHNN) Local Guidelines reproduced with kind permission from Critical Care Unit, NHNN, London, UK. (Alder, J & Malone, D 2012; Stiller, K, 2000)

Box 7.9 Stepwise approach to mobilisation

- Facilitate rolling
- Facilitate sitting up over the edge of the bed
- Hoist to chair (agree on a time limit)
- Tilt table
- Standing frame
- Sit to stand/stand to sit
- Gait
- Therabike/cardiovascular training

Adapted from Early Rehabilitation/Mobilisation in a Neurosurgical Critical Care Unit Algorithm. The National Hospital for Neurology & Neurosurgery (NHNN) Local Guidelines reproduced with kind permission from Critical Care Unit, NHNN, London, UK. (Alder, J & Malone, D 2012; Stiller, K, 2000)

RESPIRATORY TREATMENT AND MANAGEMENT
Maintenance of a Patent Airway

Patients with neurological weakness often present with an ineffective cough, resulting in sputum retention, and are at risk of recurring chest infections, hospitalisation and death. Sputum retention and atelectasis are common clinical problems (see Box 7.10) for airway clearance.

Box 7.10 When to consider airway clearance techniques

- Oxygen saturation falls below 95%;
- PCF is equal to or less than 270 L/min;
- VC falls below 1500 mL or 50% predicted value.

The maximal insufflation capacity (MIC) is the maximal volume of air that can be held in the lungs after breath stacking. The aim of MIC is to increase the inspiratory reserve volume further than the active ability of the inspiratory muscles. Key interventions are breath stacking, glossopharyngeal breathing, lung volume recruitment (LVR) bags and using the mechanical insufflation and exsufflation (MI:E) device (see Fig 7.3; see common techniques in Box 7.11). When using any adjunct with positive pressure, consideration must be given to the following contraindications:

● bulbar involvement;
● inability to protect airway (poor swallow);
● vomiting.

See key reminders to optimise treatment effects in Box 7.12.

Box 7.11 Common techniques for sputum retention and/or atelectasis (BTS/ICS 2016; Chatwin et al 2003)

● **Breath stacking**
  ○ Facilitates an increase in inspiratory volume (Bott et al 2009).
  ○ Consider regular breath stacking (10–15 maximal lung inflations three times a day).
  ○ Increases maximal insufflation capacity (MIC) (increased thoracic range of movement) in 70% of patients resulting in increased cough effectiveness (Kang & Bach 2000).
● **Glossopharyngeal breathing** (e.g. frog breathing)
  ○ A positive pressure technique that can be used to assist failing respiratory muscles, which may be useful for some patients (Maltais 2011).
● **Lung volume recruitment (LVR) bags**
  ○ LVR bags can be used as an adjunct to improve MIC.
  ○ Start by using LVR, then consider using the mechanical insufflation and exsufflation (MI:E) device.
● **Manually assisted cough (MAC)**
  ○ Involves the application of an abdominal thrust or costal lateral compression using hand placements after an adequate spontaneous inspiration or maximal insufflation.
● **Mechanical insufflation and exsufflation (MI:E) device**
  ○ Applies positive pressure to the airways, then rapidly switches to a negative pressure to stimulate the expiratory flow needed to cough and thus aid the clearance of secretions (Chatwin et al 2003).
  ○ Indicated when there is inspiratory, expiratory and bulbar dysfunction.
  ○ Assists with recruiting lung volumes, optimising thoracic range of motion and increasing lung compliance (Chatwin & Simmonds 2009).
  ○ May reduce reintubation rates (Gonçalves et al 2012).

Box 7.11 Common techniques for sputum retention and/or atelectasis (BTS/ICS 2016; Chatwin et al 2003)—cont'd

- Intermittent positive pressure breathing (IPPB)
  - Provides a patient-triggered passive inspiration which is larger than that which the patient would be able to generate by themselves.
  - Delivered via an MI:E machine or a IPPB device.
- Noninvasive ventilation (NIV)
  - The provision of ventilator support via a patient's upper airway and is often used overnight (BTS/ICS 2016).

Box 7.12 Key reminders to optimise treatment effects

- **Position**: Consider patient position.
- **Manual techniques**: Use treatment adjuncts with manual techniques, such as vibrations, to increase peak expiratory flow (Shannon et al 2010).
- **Suction:** Have suction equipment readily to hand.
- **Humidification**: Consider optimal delivery method for humidification, which improves the viscoelasticity of the sputum (BTS 2017, fphcare 2015).

Respiratory Muscle Training

Respiratory muscle weakness is common in patients with neuromuscular dysfunction resulting in:

- inadequate ventilation leading to a reduction in vital capacity and expansion of the chest wall;
- nocturnal hypoventilation;
- ineffective cough leading to sputum retention, infection and atelectasis.

Inspiratory muscle training is recommended in patients with suspected or confirmed respiratory muscle weakness (Bott et al 2009). There is inconclusive evidence to support the efficacy of inspiratory and expiratory muscle training (Van Houtte et al 2006); however, some benefit may be experienced in the neuromuscular disease and spinal cord injury population (Van Houtte et al 2006).

Management of Acute Respiratory Failure

Neurological patients in acute respiratory failure are likely to require some form of mechanical ventilation, which will be led by the medical/neurointensivist team. The aim of physiotherapy intervention is to optimise respiratory function while maintaining the neuromusculoskeletal system. Common interventions are:

- suction;
- manual techniques;
- positioning;
- manual hyperinflation (MHI)/ventilator hyperinflation (VHI);
- mobilisation.

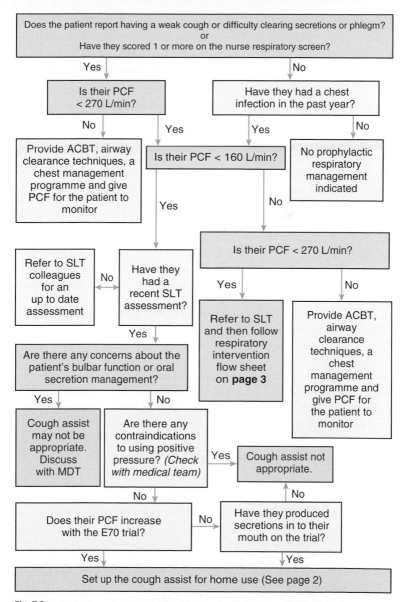

Fig. 7.3
Trial and provision of Cough Assist guideline. PCF, peak cough flow; ACBT, active cycle of breathing technique; SLT, speech and language therapist; MDT, multidisciplinary team. NHNN Local Guidelines reproduced with kind permission from Neuromuscular Complex Care Centre, NHNN, London, UK.

Tracheostomy and weaning

A tracheostomy is an artificial airway inserted directly into the trachea to facilitate ventilation and secretion clearance (see Box 7.13). Tracheostomy weaning should be through a patient, goal-centred and multidisciplinary approach (Hunt & McGowan 2015).

Box 7.13 Considerations for the insertion of a tracheostomy in patients with neurological impairment

- The inability to protect and maintain the airway
- Upper airway obstruction
- Excessive bronchial secretions
- Avoidance of laryngeal complications of prolonged ventilation
- Assist with ventilator weaning

RESPIRATORY FUNCTION IN NEUROLOGICAL CONDITIONS

The respiratory control centres (RCC) are located in the pons and medulla within the brain stem and primary set the rate, rhythm, depth and modulation of breathing. Conditions that affect these centres can have a detrimental impact on breathing and ventilation (Table 7.1).

Lesions or Conditions Affecting the Respiratory Control Centres

Subarachnoid Haemorrhage

Specific BP parameters are set by the neurosurgeon/intensive care specialist to maintain adequate cerebral perfusion. It is essential to ensure the patient has adequate pain relief before intervention. Patients must be monitored for any changes in their neurological status, for example, limb weakness, changes in conscious levels or a drop in their Glasgow Coma Score. Patients with vasospasm will usually be on a vasopressor to increase BP which should prohibit mobilisation (see Box 7.14).

Box 7.14 Interventions to be used with caution

- Coughing
- Straining (Valsalva manoeuvre)
- Manual techniques if they cause a pain response
  If vasospasm is present:
- ventilator hyperventilation (VHI);
- manual hyperinflation (MHI);
- noninvasive ventilation (NIV);
- cough assist (MI:E);
- intermittent positive pressure breathing (IPPB);
- changes in posture from supine to upright.

Table 7.1 Central nervous system conditions (Howard & Davidson 2003, Howard et al 1992, Polkey et al 1999)

Common respiratory problems in	Respiratory considerations	Treatment considerations
Unilateral or bilateral tegmental infarcts in the pons	Apneustic breathing (deep, gasping inspiration with a pause at full inspiration, followed by brief insufficient release) Impairment of carbon dioxide responsiveness	Reduced response to demands on cardiorespiratory systems during exercise Any surgical nasal approach should be treated with caution when considering any invasive nasal modality (e.g. nasal suction, IPPV)
Lateral medullary syndrome	Acute failure of automatic respiration	Requires mechanical ventilation
Basal pons infarcts Pyramids and adjacent ventral portion of the medulla	Irregular breathing pattern Inability to initiate volitional breathing	Inability to effectively cough to command Inability to breathe deeply on command Inability to hold the breath
Lesion in anterior pathways	Loss of automatic control Apnoea (cessation of breathing)	Requires mechanical ventilation

Spinal Cord Injury and Disease

Respiratory function and treatment will depend on the neurological level and whether the lesion is complete or incomplete. In the management of patients with spinal cord injury, liaison with the clinical team is essential regarding any spinal precautions that will affect physiotherapeutic treatment (Table 7.2).

Spinal injuries above the level of T6 are at risk of haemodynamic instability because of the loss of sympathetic outflow. This results in hypotension and bradycardia on suctioning. Intravenous atropine should be available.

In patients with diaphragm and respiratory muscle involvement, continuous positive airway pressure will not improve ventilation and will increase carbon dioxide retention. NIV should be considered in conjunction with the multi disciplinary team. Mechanical cough assist machines have been found to be a useful adjunct in the presence of altered or absent cough and may be useful prophylactically.

Table 7.2 Spinal cord level and respiratory function (Clapham 2004, Howard & Davidson 2003, Pryor 1999)

Level of lesion	Affected respiratory muscles	Respiratory considerations	Treatment options
C2	Diaphragm Intercostals Abdominals Accessory muscles	No respiratory effort Ventilator dependent No cough Fatigue	Suction Manual or ventilator Hyper-inflation Manual techniques Mechanical cough device Manual assisted cough
C4	Partial diaphragm Partial accessory muscles Intercostals abdominals	Ventilator independent but may require nocturnal ventilation Paradoxical breathing Ineffective cough Fatigue	Glossopharyngeal breathing Assisted cough machine Manual assisted cough Intermittent positive pressure breathing (IPPB) Mechanical cough
C6	Partial accessory muscles Intercostals Abdominals	Ventilator independent Ineffective cough Fatigue	As for C4
T1	Intercostals and abdominals	Ineffective cough Fatigue	As for C6
T12	None	Effective cough	All respiratory physiotherapy techniques

Anterior Horn Cell Conditions

Respiratory insufficiency occurs because of respiratory muscle weakness or associated bulbar weakness, leading to aspiration and bronchopneumonia (Table 7.3) (Howard & Davidson 2003).

Table 7.3 Anterior horn cell (Howard & Davidson 2003, Howard & Orwell 2002, Polkey et al 1999, Winslow & Rozovsky 2003)

Common respiratory problems in	Respiratory considerations	Treatment considerations
Poliomyelitis	Respiratory muscle weakness Fatigue	All respiratory physiotherapy interventions appropriate
Motor neurone disease	Respiratory muscle weakness Bulbar weakness Fatigue	May require ventilatory support (e.g. noninvasive ventilation) All respiratory physiotherapy interventions appropriate

Neuropathy

Respiratory insufficiency occurs because of respiratory muscle weakness or associated bulbar weakness, leading to possible respiratory failure, aspiration or bronchopneumonia (Howard & Davidson 2003, Aboussouan, L 2005). The use of vital capacity monitoring is useful in determining both deterioration and resolution of respiratory function (Table 7.4).

Neuromuscular Junction

Muscle fatigue may occur in patients with pathologies affecting the neuromuscular junction. A graded regimen of rehabilitation should be used with additional ventilatory support when rehabilitating in the early stages (Table 7.5).

Table 7.4 Neuropathy (Howard & Davidson 2003)

Common respiratory problems in	Respiratory considerations	Treatment considerations
Guillain–Barré syndrome	Primarily inspiratory muscle weakness Weakness of abdominal muscles Weakness of accessory muscles Bulbar weakness Retained secretions Aspiration pneumonia Atelectasis (collapsed lung) Fatigue	Onethird will require mechanical ventilation A drop in tidal volume of <15 mL/kg indicates the need for ventilatory support May require prolonged weaning All physiotherapy techniques appropriate

Table 7.5 Neuromuscular junction (Howard & Davidson 2003)

Common respiratory problems in	Respiratory considerations	Treatment considerations
Myasthenia gravis	Diaphragm weakness may occur with mild peripheral weakness Fatigue	Long-term ventilation All physiotherapy techniques appropriate

Muscle Conditions

Respiratory insufficiency caused by respiratory muscle weakness or associated bulbar weakness can lead to possible respiratory failure, aspiration or bronchopneumonia (Howard & Davidson 2003, Aboussouan, L 2005). Associated skeletal changes may further affect respiratory function and compliance of the chest wall (Table 7.6).

Table 7.6 Muscle (Howard & Davidson 2003, Howard et al 1993, Polkey et al 1999)

Common respiratory problems in	Respiratory considerations	Treatment considerations
Duchenne muscular dystrophy	Respiratory failure develops late Intercostal and expiratory muscle weakness Scoliosis Kyphosis Bulbar weakness Fatigue	Aspiration (the entry of secretions or foreign material into the trachea or lungs) Reduced lung compliance All physiotherapy techniques appropriate Breath stacking techniques, including lung volume recruitment (LVR) bags (McKim et al 2012).
Becker muscular dystrophy	Scoliosis Respiratory muscle weakness Fatigue	All physiotherapy techniques appropriate
Fascioscapulohumeral dystrophy	May have selective diaphragm weakness Fatigue	All physiotherapy techniques appropriate
Acid maltase deficiency	Early selective diaphragm weakness Fatigue	All physiotherapy techniques appropriate

MANAGEMENT OF TRAUMATIC BRAIN INJURY

The management of traumatic brain injury is aimed at prevention of secondary brain injury (Coles 2004, Marik 2002). Secondary damage occurs to neurones because of physiological responses after the initial injury leading to cerebral ischaemia (Marik 2002) (Table 7.7).

Normal ranges for cerebral pressure and blood flow are shown in Table 7.8.

Table 7.7 Classification of brain injury

Primary brain injury	Secondary brain injury
Focal: Disruption of brain vessels Haematoma formation Contusions Traumatic subarachnoid haemorrhage	Extracranial causes: Systemic hypotension Hypoxaemia (reduced oxygen levels) Hypercarbia (excess carbon dioxide) Disturbances of blood coagulation
Diffuse: Diffuse axonal injury	Intracranial causes: Haematoma Brain swelling Disturbances in the microvascular circulation Infection

Table 7.8 Definition and normal values relating to cerebral haemodynamics (Clapham 2004, Coles 2004)

Term	Definition	Normal range
Intracranial pressure (ICP)	Pressure within the cranial cavity	0–10 mmHg
Cerebral perfusion pressure (CPP)	The net pressure of blood flow to the brain	70–100 mmHg
Cerebral blood flow (CBF)	The amount of blood that passes through the brain per minute	50 mL/100 g/min of brain tissue

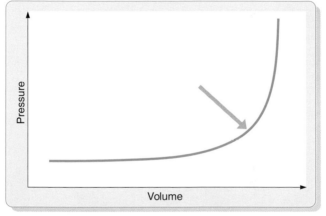

Fig. 7.4
Monro–Kellie doctrine. Graph showing the normal volume–pressure relationship within the cranial vault. The arrow indicates point where brain compliance is lost because of all compensatory mechanisms within the cranial vault being exhausted. After this point on the graph, a small rise in intracranial volume will cause an exponential rise in intracranial pressure. From Lindsay & Bone 2004, with permission.

Because of the limited space within the cranial vault, if there is a rise in volume (e.g. from a haematoma, space-occupying lesion or increase in cerebral blood volume), then there will be a subsequent rise in ICP.

In Fig. 7.4 the point marked on the curve indicates the point when the brain's compliance stops, leading to a large increase in pressure with a small increase in volume (Lindsay & Bone 2004). The signs and symptoms of raised ICP are shown in Table 7.9.

It is important for the therapist to consider any potential effects an intervention may have on cerebral perfusion pressure (CPP), as a rising ICP or a falling mean arterial pressure (MAP) can have detrimental effects which, if sustained, will lead to cerebral ischaemia (CPP = MAP − ICP). The cerebral vasculature is highly responsive to changes in the partial pressure of carbon dioxide ($Paco_2$), metabolic by-products, level of blood acidity or alkalinity and partial pressure of oxygen (PaO_2). This can result in increased cerebral blood volume, leading to an increase in ICP or cerebral ischaemia (Fig. 7.5).

Patients who have undergone a TBI commonly present with a reduced level of consciousness. Some common cardiorespiratory problems are identified in

Table 7.9 Signs and symptoms of raised intracranial pressure (ICP)

Early signs and symptoms	Late signs and symptoms
Headache	Severe headache
Confusion	Projectile vomiting
Convulsions	Reduced level of consciousness
Irritability	Irregular breathing
Lethargy	Abnormal limb posturing
Restlessness	Flexion/extension
Focal neurology	Cushing response
Pupil dysfunction	Impaired brainstem function

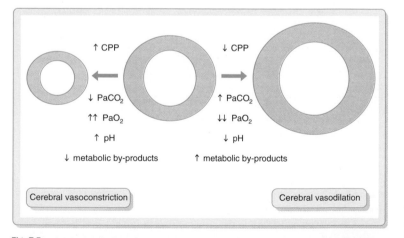

Fig. 7.5
Factors affecting cerebral vasculature. Diagram showing the effect of the reactivity of the cerebral vasculature on the partial pressure of carbon dioxide ($PaCO_2$), partial pressure of oxygen (PaO_2), blood acidity/alkalinity (pH) and metabolic by-products. CCP, cerebral perfusion pressure. From Lindsay & Bone 2004, with permission.

Table 7.10. Cardiorespiratory interventions may themselves have a detrimental effect on cerebral function; therefore a risk assessment before every respiratory intervention should be carried out involving ICP and CPP (Table 7.11).

If therapy is indicated and the risk of treatment is deemed acceptable, the potential detrimental effects associated with individual treatment modalities need to be carefully considered (Table 7.12).

Table 7.10 Common problems with reduced consciousness level (Clapham 2004, Pryor & Prasad 2008)

Common problems	Treatment considerations
Reduced airway protection	● Use of airway protection techniques
Sputum retention	● Insertion of nasopharyngeal airway (if nonintubated or had a tracheostomy [opening through the trachea to create an airway]) ● Insertion of oral airway (if nonintubated or had a tracheostomy) ● Suction ● Gravity-assisted positioning ● Manual hyperinflation ● Manual techniques, for example, chest vibrations/shaking, percussion ● Intermittent positive pressure breathing (IPPB) ● Neurophysiological facilitation of respiration techniques
Hypoventilation	● Manual hyperinflation ● IPPB ● Noninvasive ventilation (NIV)
Atelectasis (collapsed lung)	● Manual hyperventilation ● IPPB
Type II respiratory failure (low oxygen, with high carbon dioxide)	● Liaise with critical care specialist ● May require intubation or NIV

Table 7.11 Risk assessment (Clapham 2004)

Intracranial pressure (ICP)	Cerebral perfusion pressure (CPP)	Risk
<15 mmHg	70 mmHg (stable)	Low
15–20 mmHg	70 mmHg (settles quickly after treatment within 5 minutes)	Moderate
>20 mmHg	Low	High

Table 7.12 Effects of respiratory intervention (Clapham 2004, Paratz & Burns 1993, Pryor & Prasad 2008)

Physiotherapy technique	Potential treatment effects
Manual hyperinflation (MHI)/ Ventilator hyperventilation (VHI)	↑ intrathoracic pressure leading to: ↓ venous return to the heart leading to ↑ cerebral blood volume and ↑ intracranial pressure (ICP) ↓ filling pressure to the right atrium from the inferior vena cava leading to ↓ in stroke volume and drop in blood pressure The depth and rate of manual hyperventilation will affect the cerebral vasculature as a result of carbon dioxide retention or removal. This can either reduce or increase intracranial pressure. If intracranial pressure is high, then rapid, small-volume breaths will reduce ICP by removal of CO_2 to allow intermittent manual hyperinflation breaths. Intersperse this with large-volume MHI breaths for therapeutic effect.
Positioning	Treatment position may be limited to 15–30 degrees head-up position to reduce ICP. Head must be kept aligned in midline (chin in line with sternum) to reduce pooling of venous blood within the brain from neck vein obstruction in patients with a raised ICP. Patients may not tolerate turning. Bolus sedation may be required. When changing position, do so slowly in patients with raised ICP. Risk of aspiration if bulbar weakness.
Manual techniques (shaking, vibrations, percussion)	Noxious stimulation; therefore: Ensure adequate analgesia May require bolus sedation (N.B. bolus sedation may drop blood pressure) Bronchospasm Slow, single-handed percussion may reduce ICP
Intermittent positive pressure breathing (IPPB)/The Bird/ noninvasive ventilation (NIV)	↑ intrathoracic pressure therefore may have similar effects to MHI May reduce mean arterial pressure (MAP)
Suction	Hypoxia Hypercapnia leading to ↑ ICP ↑ intrathoracic pressure caused by coughing leading to increased ICP Valsalva manoeuvre (forced exhalation against closed vocal cords) Vasovagal response (cardioinhibitory and vasodepressor responses) leading to bradycardia (heart rate under 60 beats per minute)

Remember that to minimise the detrimental effects of physiotherapy intervention:
- keep treatment time short (Clapham 2004);
- increase the patient's level of sedation;
- ideally do one intervention at a time to observe how the patient responds and to assess the efficacy of the intervention.

This chapter is an abridged version adapted from Capp and Platt (2018) with permission.

References

Aboussouan, L.F., 2005. Respiratory disorders in neurologic diseases. Cleveland Clinic Journal of Medicine 72, 511–520.

Adler, J., Malone, D., 2012. Early mobilisation in the intensive care unit: a systematic review. Cardiopulmonary Physical Therapy Journal 23 (1), 5–13.

BTS/ACPRC guidelines,2009: physiotherapy management of the adult, medical, spontaneously breathing patient. Thorax 64 (Suppl. 1), i1–i51. Also available online at: www.brit-thoracic.org.uk/physioguide.

Bruton, A., 2011. Respiratory management in neurological rehabilitation. In: Stokes, M., Stack, E. (Eds.), Physical Management for Neurological Conditions. Elsevier Science, London.

BTS Guideline for oxygen therapy use in adults in healthcare and emergency settings, 2017. Thorax 72 (Supp. 1), i1–i90.

BTS/ICS, 2016. Guidelines for the ventilatory management of acute hypercapnic respiratory failure in adults. Thorax 71 (Suppl. 2), ii1–ii35.

Capp, A., Platt, L., 2018. Respiratory management (chapter 6). In: Lennon, S., Ramdharry, G., Verheyden, G. (Eds.), Physical Management for Neurological Conditions, fourth ed. Elsevier Science, London.

Chatwin, M., Ross, E., Hart, N., Nickol, A.H., Polkey, M.I., Simonds, A.K., 2003. Cough augmentation with mechanical insufflation/exsufflation in patients with neuromuscular weakness. European Respiratory Journal 21, 502–508.

Chatwin, M., Simonds, A.K., 2009. 'The addition of mechanical insufflation/exsufflation shortens airway-clearance sessions in neuromuscular patients with chest infection. Respiratory Care 54 (11), 1473–1479.

Clapham, L., 2004. Calls to the neurology/neurosurgical unit. In: Harden, B. (Ed.), Emergency Physiotherapy. Churchill Livingstone, Edinburgh.

Coles, J., 2004. Regional ischemia after head injury. Neuroscience 10, 120–125.

Gonçalves, M.R., Honrado, T., Winck, J.C., Paiva, J.A., 2012. Effects of mechanical insufflation-exsufflation in preventing respiratory failure after extubation: a randomized control trial'. Critical Care 16, R48.

Fisher & Paykel Healthcare (Fphcare), 2015. Essential humidity for a successful noninvasive ventilation strategy. Accessed at: www.fphcare.com.

Hodgson, C.L., Stiller, K., Needham, D.M., Tipping, C.J., et al., 2014. Expert consensus on safety criteria for active mobilisation of mechanically ventilated critically ill adults. Critical care 18, 658. https://doi.org/10.1186/s13054-014-0658-y.

Howard, R.S., Davidson, C., 2003. Long term ventilation in neurogenic respiratory failure. Journal of Neurology, Neurosurgery and Psychiatry 74 (Suppl. III), iii24–iii30.

Howard, R.S., Orwell, R.W., 2002. Management of motor neurone disease. Postgraduate Medical Journal 78, 736–741.

Howard, R.S., Wills, C.M., Hirsh, N.P., et al., 1992. Respiratory involvement in multiple sclerosis. Brain 115, 479–494.

Howard, R.S., Wills, C.M., Hirsh, N.P., Spencer, G.T., 1993. Respiratory involvement in primary muscle disorders: assessment and management. Quarterly Journal of Medicine 86, 175–189.

Hughes, R.A.C., Binaries, D., 1993. Acute neuromuscular respiratory paralysis. Journal of Neurology. Neurosurgery and Psychiatry 56, 334–343.

Hunt, K., McGowan, S., 2015. Tracheostomy management. BJA Education 15 (3), 149–153.

Kang Seong, Woong, Bach John, R., 2000. 'Maximum insufflation capacity. Chest 118, 61–65.

Lindsay, K., Bone, I., 2004. Neurology and Neurosurgery Illustrated. Churchill Livingstone, New York.

Main, E., Denehy, L., 2016. Cardiorespiratory Physiotherapy. Elsevier, UK.

Maltais, F., 2011. Glossopharyngeal breathing. American Journal of Respiratory Care 184, 381.

Marik, P., 2002. Management of head trauma. Chest 122 (2), 699.

McKim, D.A., Katz, S.L., Barrowman, N., Ni, A., LeBlanc, C., 2012. 'Lung Volume recruitment slows pulmonary function decline in Duchenne muscular dystrophy. Archive of Physical Medical Rehabilitation 93 (7), 1117–1122.

Paratz, J., Burns, Y., 1993. The effect of respiratory physiotherapy on intracranial pressure, mean arterial pressure, cerebral perfusion pressure and end tidal carbon dioxide in ventilated neurosurgical patients. Physiotherapy Theory and Practice 9, 3–11.

Polkey, M.I., Lyall, R.A., Moxham, J., Leigh, P.N., 1999. Respiratory aspects of neurological disease. Journal of Neurology, Neurosurgery and Psychiatry 66, 5–15.

Pryor, J., 1999. Physiotherapy for airway clearance. European Respiratory Journal 14, 141–1424.

Pryor, J.A., Prasad, A.S., 2008. Physiotherapy for Respiratory and Cardiac Problems: Adults and Paediatrics, fourth ed. Elseveier, London.

Shannon, H., Stiger, R., Gregson, R.K., Stocks, J., Main, E., 2010. Effect of chest wall vibration timing on peak expiratory flow and inspiratory pressure in a mechanically ventilated lung model. Physiotherapy 96, 344–349.

Simonds, A.K., 2016. Progress in respiratory management of bulbar complications of motor neuron disease/amyotrophic lateral sclerosis? Vol 0 No 0 1–2.

Stiller, K., 2000. Physiotherapy in intensive care. Towards an evidence based practice, Chest 118, 1801–1813.

Stiller, K., Phillips, A., 2003. Safety aspects of mobilising acutely ill inpatients. Physiotherapy Theory and Practice 19, 239–257.

Van Houtte, S., Vanlandewijk, Y., Gosselink, R., 2006. Respiratory muscle training in persons with spinal cord injury: a systemic review. Respiratory Medicine 100, 1886–1895.

West, J.B., 2012. Respiratory Physiology. The essentials, nineth ed. Lippincott Williams & Wilkins.

Winslow, C., Rozovsky, J., 2003. Effects of spinal cord injury on the respiratory system. American Journal of Physical Medicine and Rehabilitation 82 (10), 803–814.

MANAGEMENT OF COMMON CONDITIONS

CHAPTER 8

Stroke

Janne Veerbeek and Geert Verheyden

STROKE

A stroke or cerebrovascular accident (CVA) is a disorder of the central nervous system (CNS). It is defined as 'brain, spinal cord, or retinal cell death attributable to ischemia, based on: (1) pathological, imaging, or other objective evidence of cerebral, spinal cord, or retinal focal ischemic injury in a defined vascular distribution; or (2) clinical evidence of cerebral, spinal cord, or retinal focal ischemic injury based on symptoms persisting ≥24 hours or until death, and other etiologies [are] excluded' (Sacco et al 2013).

TYPES OF STROKE

There are two types of stroke: ischaemic and haemorrhagic.

- An ischaemic stroke is the result of an occluded blood vessel in the CNS caused by, for instance, a thrombosis or embolism. The majority of strokes are ischaemic (about 80%).
- A haemorrhagic stroke is the result of a ruptured blood vessel in the CNS caused by, for instance, trauma.

EPIDEMIOLOGY

- Typically affects the older population (over 65 years).
- Every 2 seconds, someone in the world has a stroke (The Stroke Association 2017).
- One in eight stroke patients dies within 30 days (The Stroke Association 2017).
- Almost two-thirds of stroke survivors leave the hospital with disability (The Stroke Association 2017).
- Worldwide, stroke is the third leading cause of disability (Murray et al 2012).

DIAGNOSIS

- Clinical assessment combined with imaging techniques, such as computed tomography (CT) or magnetic resonance imaging (MRI).

PATHOLOGY

Ischaemic stroke

● Lack of oxygen to CNS tissue after the occlusion, leading to tissue death if blood flow is not reestablished in a timely manner

Haemorrhagic stroke

● Reduced blood flow to CNS tissue after the rupture, leading to lack of oxygen

● Furthermore, compression of CNS tissue can occur from an expanding haematoma, potentially leading to additional cell death

SYMPTOMS

Stroke can lead to a wide diversity of signs and symptoms, depending on the part of the CNS that is deprived of oxygen. Possible impairments of body function are (Langhorne et al 2011):

● reduced consciousness;
● changed personality;
● lack of energy and drive;
● sleep disorders;
● reduced attention and memory;
● psychomotor and perceptual deficits;
● cognitive and visual impairments;
● altered proprioception and touch;
● change in voice and articulation;
● altered ingestion and sexuality;
● incontinence (bladder and/or bowel);
● reduced joint mobility and stability;
● loss of muscle power and endurance;
● altered muscle tone and reflexes;
● lack of control of voluntary movement;
● gait pattern dysfunctions.

PROGNOSIS

Generally, most recovery is observed in the first month poststroke, with further recovery (but at a slower rate) happening up until 3 months, from which point there is a stagnation of recovery (Langhorne et al 2011, Verheyden et al 2008).

Established predictors for better activities of daily living (ADLs) independency at 3 months and beyond are (Kwakkel & Kollen 2013, Veerbeek et al 2011):

● younger age;
● less severe stroke deficit;
● better sitting balance;

- no urinary continence;
- limited comorbidity;
- conscious at admission;
- better cognitive status;
- absence of depression.

For regaining independent walking at 6 months, confirmed prognostic variables are (Kwakkel & Kollen 2013):

- younger age;
- less severe motor impairment of the paretic leg;
- absence of homonymous hemianopia;
- no urinary continence;
- better sitting balance;
- better initial ADL and ambulation;
- better level of consciousness on admission.

When predicting upper limb outcome up until 6 months, recognised variables of better outcome are (Coupar et al 2012, Nijland et al 2010):

- less severe initial motor impairment of the paretic arm (e.g. presence of shoulder abduction and finger extension);
- integrity of the corticospinal tract.

MEDICAL MANAGEMENT

Time is brain. The more rapidly the blood flow is restored to the CNS tissue affected, the fewer nerve cells die (Saver 2006).

Core (hyper)acute medical stroke management includes:

- For ischaemic stroke, the obstructed blood vessel can be targeted by means of clot-busting medication (thrombolysis) within 4.5 hours poststroke. Furthermore, a blood clot can be mechanically removed by means of thrombectomy, which entraps the blood clot by a device inserted through an artery and subsequently withdrawn from the body.
- In case of haemorrhagic stroke, stopping the bleeding in the brain is crucial, and some patients require neurosurgical intervention to achieve this. Increased intracranial pressure can be reduced by a craniotomy.
- People after stroke should be admitted to a dedicated acute stroke unit where an interdisciplinary team with specialists in stroke care monitors the patient.

ASSESSMENT

Irrespective of the stage poststroke – hyperacute (0–24 hours), acute (1–7 days), early subacute (7 days–3 months), late subacute (3–6 months), and chronic (>6 months) (Bernhardt et al 2017) – patient-related characteristics as well as standardised measurement tools should be collected to document the patient's status (Table 8.1). The frequency of assessment will vary according to the phase, for example, daily in the (hyper)acute, weekly in the early subacute, monthly in the late subacute, and every 3 or 6 months in the chronic phase.

Table 8.1 Key assessment information for people with stroke

Database
Patient-specific details, including: ● Contact details ● Age ● Diagnosis ● Medical history ● Prestroke functioning ● Psychosocial, social and family status ● Home/living situation, including presence of existing adaptations ● Preferred hand
Subjective
Description of what happened at the time of stroke and since that event. Collect information from partner/relatives if communication is difficult because of speech and/or language problems or disorders of consciousness. Ask what the primary and secondary aims of the patient are to determine short- and long-term goals together with the interdisciplinary team involved.
Objective
In the (hyper)acute phase, monitor vital signs for medical stability. When patient is medically stable, use clinical observation and standardised measurement tools to objectively evaluate: ● Upper and lower limb function ● Upper limb activities ● Bed mobility ● Sit-to-stand, stand-to-sit and sit-to-sit (transfers) ● Sitting and standing balance ● Gait ● Physical fitness Integrate other measurement tools at the body function level, such as muscle tone and sensation (when relevant).
Stroke-Specific Tools
Examples of standardised measurement tools include (Langhorne et al 2011): For body functions: ● National Institutes of Health Stroke Scale (stroke severity) ● Motricity Index for upper and lower limb (muscle strength) ● Fugl–Meyer Assessment (motor impairment) ● Hospital Anxiety and Depression Scale (anxiety and depression)

Table 8.1 Key assessment information for people with stroke—cont'd

Database
For activities: ● Barthel Index (basic activities of daily living [ADL]) ● Functional Independence Measure (basic ADL) ● Berg Balance Scale (basic balance) ● Rivermead Mobility Index (basic mobility) ● 10-Metre Walk Test (gait speed) ● Action Research Arm Test (upper limb activities) ● Caregiver Strain Index (caregiver burden)
For participation: ● Nottingham Extended Activities of Daily Living (extended ADL) ● Stroke Impact Scale 3.0 (disease impact) ● Euroqol-5D (quality of life)

REHABILITATION

In the (hyper)acute phase, early interdisciplinary management aims are:

● monitoring vital signs for medical stability;
● maintaining respiratory function;
● appropriate skin care;
● positioning;
● monitoring muscle length and range of motion;
● initiating early mobilisation (i.e. bring the patient in a sitting or standing position and stimulate being physically active when medically stable, preferably by providing shorter but more frequent sessions) (Bernhardt et al 2016).

In the acute and subacute phases, emphasis is on (Langhorne et al 2011):

● restoring impairments to regain activities (days to weeks);
● task-oriented practice with adaptive learning and compensation strategies (days to months);
● specific rehabilitation interventions to improve extended ADL and social interaction (days to months);
● environmental adaptations and services at home (weeks to months).

In the chronic phase, the focus is on maintenance of mobility and physical condition and monitoring quality of life.

PHYSIOTHERAPY INTERVENTIONS

General recommendations for stroke physiotherapy that are assumed to determine effectiveness of motor learning are exercises that are (KNGF-guideline Stroke 2014; for selected interventions see Table 8.2):

● tailored to the individual;
● include repetition, but with variations;

Table 8.2 Key stroke interventions for motor rehabilitation for which the best evidence is available

Lower Limb and Locomotor Therapy	
Intervention	**Description**
Balance training	<ul><li>Exercises aimed at maintaining, achieving or restoring a state of balance during any posture (Pollock et al 2014). Training should include various postures and, if possible, walking.</li><li>Positive effects on sitting and standing balance and basic activities of daily living (ADL) (Van Duijnhoven et al 2016, Veerbeek et al 2014).</li><li>Recommended duration: 4–6 weeks, 2–7 times/week, 15–60 minutes/session (KNGF-guideline Stroke 2014).</li></ul>
Overground walking	<ul><li>Therapy without technological equipment, allowing and stimulating walking over a regular even surface.</li><li>Beneficial effects on walking speed and walking distance (States et al 2009). To be provided to both walkers and nonwalkers.</li><li>Recommended duration: 2–6 months, 1–5 times/week, 15–60 minutes/session (KNGF-guideline Stroke 2014).</li></ul>
Speed-dependent treadmill training	<ul><li>The patient walks on a treadmill, eventually with support of one or both upper limbs. A therapist can facilitate walking if needed.</li><li>Significant improvements for gait speed and width of the gait pattern (Mehrholz et al 2014, Veerbeek et al 2014). Suggested for walkers only.</li><li>Recommended duration: 2 weeks–6 months, 3–5 times/week, 8–60 minutes/session (KNGF-guideline Stroke 2014).</li></ul>
Body weight–supported treadmill training	<ul><li>Patients walk on a treadmill with partial body-weight support from a harness fixed above the patient's head. Percentage of body weight supported is gradually reduced.</li><li>Positive effects on comfortable walking speed and walking distance (Mehrholz et al 2014, Veerbeek et al 2014). Suggested for dependent walkers.</li><li>Recommended duration: 2–6 weeks, 3–6 times/week, 15–90 minutes/session (KNGF-guideline Stroke 2014).</li></ul>
Robot-assisted gait training	<ul><li>Patient's walking is guided by electromechanically guiding footplates and/or orthoses, with the patient secured through a harness.</li><li>Beneficial effects on walking speed, walking distance, heart rate, balance, walking ability and basic ADL (Mehrholz et al 2013; Veerbeek et al 2014). Suggested for dependent walkers.</li><li>Recommended duration: 2–10 weeks, 3–7 times/week, 15–60 minutes/session (KNGF-guideline Stroke 2014).</li></ul>

Table 8.2 Key stroke interventions for motor rehabilitation for which the best evidence is available—cont'd

Lower Limb and Locomotor Therapy	
Intervention	Description
Circuit class training	● A group of patients independently practice through a number of workstations under the supervision of a limited number of therapists. ● Significant improvements in walking speed, walking distance, balance, walking ability and physical activity (Veerbeek et al 2014). However, task specificity of the exercises is important, that is, patients should practice what was formulated to be the treatment goal (English et al 2015). ● Recommended duration: 4–19 weeks, 3–5 times/week, 30–75 minutes/session (KNGF-guideline Stroke 2014).
Electrostimulation	● Adding neuromuscular stimulation (NMS) when performing a functional task or when performing nonfunctional movements of the affected lower limb. ● Positive effects on motor function, muscle strength and resistance to passive movements (Veerbeek et al 2014). ● Optimal settings are unknown.
Upper Limb Therapy	
Constraint-induced movement therapy (CIMT)	● Two- to three-week approach to stimulate involvement of affected upper limb by (1) repetitive, task-oriented, progressive upper limb training for 6 hours per day; (2) wearing a mitt on the less affected hand for 90% of the waking hours; and (3) provision of a transfer package stimulating learned use into the patient's daily life (Morris et al 2006). Modifications of CIMT typically include a lower number of training hours a day, but therapy is provided over a longer period. ● Beneficial effects on upper limb activities and patient-reported daily life upper limb use (Kwakkel et al 2015, Veerbeek et al 2014). ● CIMT is for a selected group of patients only, that is, those with voluntary extension movement in one or more fingers of the affected hand.
Virtual reality (including interactive video gaming)	● Defined as 'the use of interactive simulations created with computer hardware and software to present users with opportunities to engage in environments that appear and feel similar to real world objects and events' (Weiss et al 2006). ● Significant improvements for basic ADL, but muscle tone should be assessed, as the literature suggests a potential increase in tone of the paretic upper limb (Veerbeek et al 2014). ● Recommended duration: several weeks, 5 times/week, 30 minutes/session (KNGF-guideline Stroke 2014).

8

Continued

Table 8.2 Key stroke interventions for motor rehabilitation for which the best evidence is available—cont'd

Upper Limb Therapy	
Intervention	Description
Electrostimulation	● Adding NMS or electromyography-triggered NMS (EMG-NMS) when performing a functional task or when performing nonfunctional movements of the affected upper limb. ● Positive effects on motor function and for EMG-NMS, additional positive effects on upper limb activities (Veerbeek et al 2014). ● Optimal settings are unknown.
Robot-assisted therapy	● With mechanical devices using electronic, computerised control systems, patients train their affected upper limb. The devices can provide movement, movement assistance or resistance. ● Significant but small improvement in upper limb motor function (Mehrholz et al 2015, Veerbeek et al 2017), with a potentially increased risk for developing higher upper limb muscle tone. ● Optimal settings are unknown and indication remains speculative.

For a more detailed description see Veerbeek & Verheyden 2018.

● comprise rest periods between sessions and repetitions;
● include feedback on performance and results;
● motivational for the patient by providing information about the goal of the exercise;
● offered fragmented at first (in the case of complex movements, e.g. dressing) but practiced as a whole in the case of automatised movements (e.g. walking);
● conducted in a meaningful environment.

This chapter is an abridged version adapted from Veerbeek and Verheyden (2018) with permission.

References

Bernhardt, J., Churilov, L., Ellery, F., Collier, J., Chamberlain, J., Langhorne, P., et al., 2016. Prespecified dose-response analysis for A Very Early Rehabilitation Trial (AVERT). Neurology 86 (23), 2138–2145.

Bernhardt, J., Hayward, K.S., Kwakkel, G., Ward, N.S., Wolf, S.L., Borschmann, K., Krakauer, J.W., Boyd, L.A., Carmichael, S.T., Corbett, D., Cramer, S.C., 2017. Agreed definitions and a shared vision for new standards in stroke recovery research: The Stroke Recovery and Rehabilitation Roundtable taskforce. International Journal of Stroke 12 (5), 444–450.

Coupar, F., Pollock, A., Rowe, P., Weir, C., Langhorne, P., 2012. Predictors of upper limb recovery after stroke: a systematic review and meta-analysis. Clinical Rehabilitation 26 (4), 291–313.

English, C., Bernhardt, J., Crotty, M., Esterman, A., Segal, L., Hillier, S., 2015. Circuit class therapy or seven-day week therapy for increasing rehabilitation intensity of therapy after stroke (CIRCIT): a randomized controlled trial. International Journal of Stroke 10 (4), 594–602.

KNGF-guideline Stroke. 2014. https://www.fysionet-evidencebased.nl/index.php/kngf-guidelines-in-english. [Accessed 27 May 2017].

Kwakkel, G., Kollen, B.J., 2013. Predicting activities after stroke: what is clinically relevant? International Journal of Stroke 8 (1), 25–32.

Kwakkel, G., Veerbeek, J.M., Van Wegen, E.E., Wolf, S.L., 2015. Constraint-induced movement therapy after stroke. Lancet Neurology 14 (2), 224–234.

Langhorne, P., Bernhardt, J., Kwakkel, G., 2011. Stroke rehabilitation. Lancet 377 (9778), 1693–1702.

Mehrholz, J., Elsner, B., Werner, C., Kugler, J., Pohl, M., 2013. Electromechanical-assisted training for walking after stroke. Cochrane Database of Systematic Reviews (7), CD006185.

Mehrholz, J., Pohl, M., Elsner, B., 2014. Treadmill training and body weight support for walking after stroke. Cochrane Database of Systematic Reviews (1), CD002840.

Mehrholz, J., Pohl, M., Platz, T., Kugler, J., Elsner, B., 2015. Electromechanical and robot-assisted arm training for improving activities of daily living, arm function, and arm muscle strength after stroke. Cochrane Database of Systematic Reviews (11), CD006876.

Morris, D.M., Taub, E., Mark, V.W., 2006. Constraint-induced movement therapy: characterizing the intervention protocol. Europa Medicophysica 42 (3), 257–268.

Murray, C.J., Vos, T., Lozano, R., Naghavi, M., et al., 2012. Disability-adjusted life years (DALYs) for 291 diseases and injuries in 21 regions, 1990-2010: a systematic analysis for the Global Burden of Disease Study 2010. Lancet 380 (9859), 2197–2223.

Nijland, R.H., Van Wegen, E.E., Harmeling-Van der Wel, B.C., Kwakkel, G., EPOS Investigators, 2010. Presence of finger extension and shoulder abduction within 72 hours after stroke predicts functional recovery. Early prediction of functional outcome after stroke: the EPOS cohort study. Stroke 41 (4), 745–750.

Pollock, A., Baer, G., Campbell, P., Choo, P.L., Forster, A., Morris, J., Pomeroy, V.M., Langhorne, P., 2014. Physical rehabilitation approaches for the recovery of function and mobility following stroke. Cochrane Database of Systematic Reviews (4), CD001920.

Sacco, R.L., Kasner, S.E., Broderick, J.P., Caplan, L.R., American Heart Association Stroke Council, Council on Cardiovascular Surgery and Anaesthesia, et al., 2013. An updated definition of stroke for the 21st century: a statement for healthcare professionals from the American Heart Association/American Stroke Association. Stroke 44 (7), 2064–2089.

Saver, J.L., 2006. Time is brain – quantified. Stroke 37 (1), 263–266.

States, R.A., Pappas, E., Salem, Y., 2009. Overground physical therapy gait training for chronic stroke patients with mobility deficits. Cochrane Database of Systematic Reviews (3), CD006075.

8

The Stroke Association, January 2017. State of the Nation: stroke statistics. https://www. stroke.org.uk/sites/default/files/state_of_the_nation_2017_final_1.pdf. [Accessed 2 March 2017].

Van Duijnhoven, H.J., Heeren, A., Peters, M.A., Veerbeek, J.M., Kwakkel, G., Geurts, A.C., et al., 2016. Effects of exercise therapy on balance capacity in chronic stroke: systematic review and meta-analysis. Stroke 47 (10), 2603–2610.

Veerbeek, J.M., Kwakkel, G., Van Wegen, E.E., Ket, J.C., Heymans, M.W., 2011. Early prediction of outcome of activities of daily living after stroke: a systematic review. Stroke 42 (5), 1482–1488.

Veerbeek, J.M., Van Wegen, E., Van Peppen, R., Van der Wees, P.J., Hendriks, E., Rietberg, M., Kwakkel, G., 2014. What is the evidence for physical therapy poststroke? A systematic review and meta-analysis. PLoS One 9 (2), e87987.

Veerbeek, J.M., Langbroek-Amersfoort, A.C., Van Wegen, E.E., Meskers, C.G., Kwakkel, G., 2017. Effects of robot-assisted therapy for the upper limb after stroke. Neurorehabil Neural Repair 31 (2), 107–121.

Veerbeek, J.M., Verheyden, G.S.A.F., 2018. Stroke. In: Lennon, S., Ramdharry, G., Verheyden, G. (Eds.), Physical Management for Neurological Conditions, fourth ed. Elsevier, London.

Verheyden, G., Nieuwboer, A., De Wit, L., Thijs, V., Dobbelaere, J., Devos, H., et al., 2008. Time course of trunk, arm, leg, and functional recovery after ischemic stroke. Neurorehabil Neural Repair 22 (2), 173–179.

Weiss, P., Kizony, R., Feintuch, U., Katz, N., 2006. Virtual reality in neurorehabilitation. In: Selzer, M., Cohen, L., Gage, F., Clarke, S., Duncan, P. (Eds.), Textbook of Neural Repair and Rehabilitation. Cambridge University Press.

CHAPTER 9

Traumatic brain injury

Gavin Williams

INTRODUCTION

Traumatic brain injury (TBI) is a particular type of acquired brain injury (ABI) that describes a single-event injury to the brain caused by an external force. TBI remains the primary cause of death and disability for young adults. The primary causes of TBI are motor vehicle accidents, falls, sporting accidents and assaults.

EPIDEMIOLOGY

- Highest incidence is in adolescents and younger adults aged 15 to 45 years, primarily caused by road trauma and sport-related concussions.
- Males are almost three times more likely to be injured and to have more severe injuries.
- Approximately 200 to 300 new cases present for medical evaluation per 100,000 population each year.
- Falls and head strikes are a major cause of head trauma in children under the age of 2 years and in older adults aged over 75 years.
- The terms *concussion* and *mild TBI* are often used interchangeably, and full recovery is expected in 80% to 90% of cases within 7 to 10 days (McCrory et al 2013). The Sport Concussion Assessment Tool version 5 (SCAT5) is the recommended assessment tool for concussion/mild TBI (Echemendia et al 2017).

PATHOPHYSIOLOGY

- TBI typically occurs as a result of a high-velocity, high-impact blow to the head, most commonly caused by road trauma and falls (O'Connor 2002, O'Connor & Cripps 1999).
- The primary injury is associated with the mechanical forces acting on the brain which result in a combination of acceleration, deceleration and rotational forces (Crooks et al 2007).
- The initial injury response leads to oedema which, in conjunction with contusion, hematomas and haemorrhage, causes additional compressive forces, which can further disturb brain function by distorting brain tissue, elevating intracranial pressure (ICP) or reducing cerebral blood flow (secondary injury).

Table 9.1 Key features associated with primary and secondary brain injury

Primary injury	Secondary injury
● Occurs at the time of injury ● Closed or blunt injury ● Open or penetrating injury ● Contrecoup movement Cerebral contusion as the brain collides with the inside of the skull, moving back and forth within the skull, producing further shearing damage. ● Diffuse axonal injury (Crooks et al 2007) The neuronal injury associated with contrecoup movement and rotational forces. ● Haemorrhages	● Occurs after the initial impact ● Disrupted autoregulation ● Compression ● Reduced blood flow ● Elevated intracranial pressure ● Hypoxia ● Hypotension

● Orthopaedic, chest, spinal, abdominal and limb injuries are common associated injuries (Table 9.1).

DIAGNOSIS

● Initial diagnosis is based on factors such as orientation, arousal or conscious state. In the majority of cases, TBI is associated with a period of loss of consciousness.

● The severity of TBI ranges from mild concussion with transient symptoms to very severe injury resulting in death assessed by loss of consciousness or coma (depth and duration) and posttraumatic amnesia (PTA).

● Coma is defined as 'not obeying commands, not uttering words and not opening eyes'; it is usually measured by the Glasgow Coma Scale (GCS) (Teasdale & Jennett 1974).

● PTA is the period of time from the accident until the person is orientated to their surroundings. The Galveston Orientation and Amnesia Test (GOAT) (Levin et al 1979) and the Westmead PTA scale (Shores et al 1986) are among the most widely used measures of length of PTA (Tables 9.2 and 9.3).

Table 9.2 TBI severity: Glasgow Coma Score (GCS) depth and duration (Bond 1986, 1990)

GCS classification	Depth (scored in first 24 hr)	Duration of GCS ≤8
Mild	13–15	<15 min
Moderate	9–12	15 min – 6 hr
Severe	3–8	6–48 hr
Very Severe		>48 hr

Table 9.3 Traumatic brain injury: severity and duration of posttraumatic amnesia (PTA) (Shores et al 1986)

Severity of injury	Duration of PTA
Very Mild	<5 min
Mild	5–60 min
Moderate	<24 hr
Severe	1–6 days
Very Severe	7–28 days
Extremely Severe	>28 days

MEDICAL MANAGEMENT

Early management interventions, including immediate resuscitation and early intubation, rapid admission to a dedicated trauma unit, early scanning and evacuation of intracranial haematomas and monitoring of ICP, have significantly improved mortality and morbidity (Table 9.4) (Bragge et al 2015). See Carney et al (2017) for an overview of the medical and surgical management of TBI.

Management of moderate to severe trauma cases involves a large team of specialists and is a particularly stressful time for the patient's family and friends. Additional

Table 9.4 Guiding principles for acute management (Carney et al 2017)

Clinical problem	Recommended management
Intracranial pressure (ICP)	● Management of severe traumatic brain injury patients using information from ICP monitoring is recommended (>20 mmHg)
Infection	● Increased risk of infection arising from interventions such as ICP monitoring and intubation. ● Prophylactic antibiotics are no longer recommended for intubation to reduce the risk of pneumonia or external ventricular drains
Deep venous thrombosis (DVT)	● Compression stockings are recommended prophylactically ● Blood-thinning agents are no longer recommended for prophylactic management of DVT
Metabolism	● Recommendations for timing and method feeding, but not glycemic control or vitamins and supplements
Seizures	● Prophylactic use of antiseizure medication is not recommended for preventing seizures after the first 7 days

injuries associated with the mechanism of injury, such as fractures, dislocations and amputations, also need to be assessed and treated as the medical status of the patient allows. Another important goal at this stage is to prevent or monitor the development of secondary complications. The combination of a prolonged period of unconsciousness and associated bed rest, fractures, muscle paresis, spasticity and hypertonicity mean that the patient is at high risk of developing contractures and pressure areas. See Box 9.1 & 9.2 for aims & team care.

● Patients are often ventilated, sedated, paralysed and intubated during the acute phase. This is done initially to minimise agitation caused by the negative cascade of effects of agitation leading to raised blood pressure, raised ICP and reduced brain oxygenation.

● Oxygen is usually provided (via nasal prongs or face mask) even when ventilation is not required to help meet the injured brain's increased energy requirements.

● Neurosurgery may be required in open or penetrating TBI to remove debris and clean the wound. Decompressive craniectomy, the removal of a bone flap from the skull, is required for some severe cases of raised ICP.

● ICP (>20 mmHg):

  ● The two standard interventions for the treatment of raised ICP are mannitol and hypertonic saline (Bratton et al 2007a).

  ● A slightly raised head position (avoiding neck flexion) is usually recommended for raised ICP.

  ● Usual respiratory care interventions, such as postural drainage or manual hyperinflation, may be contraindicated or used with caution, because of the associated rise in ICP (Bratton et al 2007b).

Box 9.1 Aims of acute management

● Stabilise the patient; maintain life
● Prevent further/secondary neurological damage; keep brain oxygenated
● Limit/cease bleeding
● Monitor intracranial pressure and conscious state
● Prevent complications; prevent respiratory problems (prevention of sputum retention; optimisation of lung volume; ensuring adequate ventilation)
● Preserve the integrity of the musculoskeletal system
● Improve level of consciousness
● Manage other chest, abdominal and musculoskeletal injuries

During this early stage of recovery, physiotherapy assessment for respiratory and musculoskeletal health is important, although sessions are typically short and frequent:

● Respiratory physiotherapy (Capp & Platt 2018). Injury to the brainstem can directly affect the respiratory control centres. The relationship between brain function and lung function is critical, as the brain requires adequate oxygenation to function, and the respiratory system relies on drive from the brain to control ventilation. Changes in blood gas chemistry can lead to changes within the cerebral vasculature, which can lead to brain hypoxia and secondary brain injury. It is important for the therapist to consider any potential effects an intervention may have on cerebral perfusion pressure (CPP), as a rising ICP or a falling mean arterial pressure (MAP) can have detrimental effects which, if sustained, will lead to cerebral ischaemia (CPP = MAP − ICP).

● It is critical to identify any threats to soft tissue extensibility and skin integrity. Frequent repositioning every 2 to 4 hours may help prevent musculoskeletal contractures and pressure areas on the skin.

● When a patient has a reduced level of consciousness (Table 9.5), with minimal movement and activity to command, physiotherapists use interventions such as positioning, assisted movement, serial splinting or casting and tilt-tabling in an attempt to maintain range of motion and encourage movement.

● The acute hospital environment is busy and noisy and often lit throughout the 24-hour period. It may be necessary to limit rather than increase sensory stimulation. It is important for this concept of regulated sensory stimulation to be imparted to friends and family members so they may contribute appropriately to the promotion of recovery.

Box 9.2 Common team goals during the acute phase

● Ongoing (daily) assessment
● Monitoring of respiratory status
● Prevention of contractures and pressure areas – consider interventions such as positioning and assisted movement, splinting or casting and tilt-tabling
● Liaising within the multidisciplinary team to ensure a coordinated approach
● Graded sensory stimulation
● Introduction of antigravity activity such as sitting on the edge of the bed, sitting out of bed or standing on a tilt-table
● Provision of information, education and support for family and friends

Table 9.5 Disorders of consciousness

Level of consciousness	Definition/description
Posttraumatic amnesia (PTA)	Not a true disorder of arousal. PTA is characterised by disorientation to time, person and place (Shores et al 1986).
Vegetative state (VS) or persistent vegetative state (PVS)	A clinical condition of complete unawareness of the self and the environment, accompanied by sleep–wake cycles with either complete or partial preservation of hypothalamic and brainstem automatic functions (Seel et al 2010). This state is sometimes referred to as unresponsive wakefulness syndrome (UWS).
Minimally conscious state (MCS)	A condition of severely altered consciousness in which minimal but definite behavioural evidence of self or environmental awareness is demonstrated (Giacino et al 2002). One or more of four diagnostic criteria confirm MCS and include (1) following simple commands, (2) yes/no responses, (3) intelligible verbalisation and (4) purposeful behaviour.
'Locked in' syndrome	Normal consciousness and sleep–wake cycle; preserved auditory, visual and emotional function; but limited verbal communication and bodily movement (American Congress of Rehabilitation 1995).
Coma	No verbal response, no obeying commands and the patient does not open the eyes either spontaneously or to any stimulus (Jennett & Teasdale 1977).

CLINICAL PRESENTATION

- The range and severity of the presenting signs and symptoms can be diverse because of the variability in location of focal brain injury and the extent of diffuse and secondary brain injury.
- Not all impairments are observable immediately after injury, and some psychosocial, cognitive, behavioural, emotional and sensorimotor impairments may take time to be revealed as a patient's conscious state improves and their environment changes.
- Because of the high-velocity/high-impact nature of the injury, it is not uncommon for people who sustain a TBI to have a range of other musculoskeletal, chest and abdominal injuries.

PROGNOSIS/TIME COURSE

- The key initial factor in determining survival is the immediate arrival to a trauma or emergency management unit to limit or reduce the impact of secondary brain injury (Jeremitsky et al 2003).

- The GCS and PTA scores have been used in many TBI outcome studies to predict outcome.
- Other than severity of injury, other factors that may influence outcome after TBI are:
  - Age – those who are younger tend to have better outcomes (Perrin et al 2015);
  - Cognitive reserve – those who have higher levels of premorbid cognitive function may have greater 'reserve' capacity and therefore may better cope with some levels of cognitive impairment (Schonberger et al 2011);
  - Gender – some females may have better outcomes than males (de Guise et al 2014).
- Outcome is determined by a range of factors such as independence in self-care and mobility, ability to work or study, community participation, relationships and quality of life.
- A key factor that affects TBI outcome is the support of family and friends. Up to 85% of people with moderate to severe TBI do not return to preaccident activities (Ponsford et al 1995), so a strong network of family and friends who are able to assist on a daily basis is important.
- Recovery from TBI is notoriously slow. Ongoing improvement can occur and has been documented for years after TBI, but the majority of recovery does occur by 6 months postinjury (Jennett et al 1981), with little overall change found when routinely assessed for many years (Ponsford 2014).
- Intensive rehabilitation has been shown to improve people's outcomes after TBI (Turner-Stokes et al 2016). Guidelines for postacute care are available for the United States (State of Colorado 2013), the UK (Scottish Intercollegiate Guidelines Network (SIGN) 2013) and New Zealand (New Zealand Guidelines Group 2006).

ASSESSMENT

After the initial lifesaving and subsequent brain-saving phase, the rehabilitation phase commences as the patient becomes medically stable. Careful handling is required when assessing patients who are unable to communicate pain, are in a minimally conscious state, are paretic and hypotonic or are restless or agitated. A full assessment cannot necessarily be performed in a single session or by a single therapist.

- **Cognition/perception**

  Because of the considerable impact of TBI on cognition, which in turn affects personal, domestic and community activities of daily living, a thorough cognitive or neuropsychological assessment is required (Ponsford et al 2013).

- **Behavioural problems** (Wilson 2018)

  Behavioural problems can directly interfere with therapy engagement and compliance, such as verbal or physical aggression; the use of inappropriate/

disinhibited language throughout therapy; or kicking, biting and scratching directed towards staff. The implementation of behaviour modification management is a team effort. See Box 9.3.

Box 9.3 Common emotional-behavioural difficulties after ABI (Brown 2012)

- Apathy (46%)
- Depression (20%–40%)
- Anxiety (10%–25%)
- Pain (>50%): headaches, spasticity, contractures, heterotopic ossification, complex regional pain syndromes
- Reduced anger control, posttraumatic stress disorder (19%–26%)
- Reduced community involvement
- Reduced relationship satisfaction and quality
- Inability to return to work or previously enjoyed leisure pursuits
- Severe behavioural disorders (verbal, physical and sexual disinhibition, aggression)

- The clinical presentation may fluctuate from day to day or change over time as things improve (conscious state) or develop (heterotrophic ossification [HO]) over time.
- Hypertonicity and spasticity can develop very quickly, particularly in the more severe cases (Brashear & Elovic 2010). The arms and legs may be held in decerebrate (arms and legs in extension, hands clenched) or decorticate (arms in flexion and legs in extension) postures, making active or passive movement virtually impossible.
- Muscle paresis is one of the key negative features associated with the upper motor neurone syndrome (UMNS), along with impaired coordination, motor control and fatigue (Ivanhoe & Reistetter 2004).
- Reduced muscle and joint range of motion (ROM) are primarily caused by hypertonicity and spasticity, a prolonged period of rest in bed, concurrent musculoskeletal injuries or a combination of all or some of these.
- Exaggerated muscle tendon reflexes.
- Reduced motor control.
- Dyspraxia.
- Ataxia.
- Balance and vestibular dysfunction.
- Pain may be associated with spasms, spasticity or hypertonicity or associated injuries. Injury to the brain itself can also cause pain such as central

Table 9.6 Common assessment tools in traumatic brain injury

Impairment	Common assessment tools
Hypertonicity	● Ashworth scale (AS) (Ashworth 1964) ● Modified Ashworth scale (MAS) (Bohannon & Smith 1987)
Spasticity	● Modified Tardieu scale (MTS) (Haugh et al 2006)
Weakness	● Manual muscle testing (MMT) (Morris et al 2004) ● Handheld dynamometry (Stark et al 2011)
Reduced voluntary movement	● Stroke Rehabilitation Assessment of Movement (STREAM) (Daley et al 1999)
Balance dysfunction	● Function In Sitting Test (FIST) (Gorman et al 2010) ● Berg Balance Scale (BBS) (Berg et al 1989)
Loss of range of motion (ROM)	● Goniometry

poststroke pain syndrome (Flaster et al 2013). In a subset of these patients, some may develop complex regional pain syndrome (Birklein 2005). Common assessment tools are presented in Table 9.6.

INTERVENTIONS

Important physical outcomes can be achieved for many years after TBI. Some people will be unable to return home and require assisted living. Given the complex nature of TBI, a team approach is vital. However, fragmented service delivery is common and leads to suboptimal outcomes, especially once patients return to live in the community. Service provision and evaluation of interventions in the rehabilitation phase require much further development so that support for patients and their families become more accessible and available in the longer term.

Cognitive, behavioural and emotional impairments have a major impact on how physical interventions are delivered, and independent practice may never be possible for some. A person with a TBI may be highly motivated but fail to benefit from their prescribed exercise programme because of poor memory (forgetting to do their exercises unprompted), poor initiation (lack of internal drive), poor self-monitoring (difficulty discriminating between good and poor performance) or fear or anxiety (worried about falling when walking).

● **Hypertonicity and spasticity management** Hypertonicity and spasticity medications include baclofen, dantrolene sodium, diazepam, tizanidine and botulinum toxin (BoNT-A). BoNT-A is very effective at reducing focal spasticity; however, the impact on function or activity limitations is yet to be established (Olver et al 2010, Sheean et al 2010). Most commonly, the medical management of spasticity is supported by a range of interventions provided by physiotherapists, which include stretching, casting, splinting, tilt-tabling, strength training and functional retraining.

- **Maintaining and improving ROM** Physical interventions are frequently used in conjunction with other treatments such as BoNT-A or baclofen. Maintenance of a plantargrade foot position is an important factor in achieving sitting and standing positions and walking.

  - **Serial casting:** Commonly applied to the distal joints of the arms (elbow, wrists and hands) and legs (knees and ankles) (Verplancke et al 2005, Singer et al 2003). Left in place for 7 to 10 days until being removed and a new one applied in a better (more stretched) position.

  - **Splints:** Easily modified to accommodate improvement as the stretching takes effect. Some splints are 'static' (i.e. they do not move and restrict the person from moving). Other splints are 'dynamic' (i.e. they allow movement while in situ). Can be removed for showering and dressing or to perform other exercises during therapy. Monitor carefully for pressure areas.

  - **Tilt table:** Gives a graded body-weight stretch of the calf muscles at a stage in rehabilitation when the patient is unlikely to be able to unable to stand independently. Inclination can be adjusted according to the person's physiological response, particularly when someone has been minimally conscious or in bed for a prolonged period.

- **Strength training** Strength training is safe and effective for improving muscle weakness associated with UMNS; however, as with the treatment of many physical impairments, the translation of improved muscle strength to improved function is less well established (Taylor et al 2005, Williams et al 2014). Strength training should be targeted towards the key muscle groups responsible for improved function to optimise the translation to functional gain (Williams et al 2014).

- **Task practice and function** Functional practice, or task practice, provides the opportunity to 'bring it all together' to improve performance and reduce activity limitations. Improvement in physical impairments does not necessarily automatically lead to improved participation rates (Sullivan & Cen 2011); therefore task or functional practice is the vital link in ensuring that rehabilitation outcomes are used in day-to-day life.

  - **Context:** This means that rather than just practicing activities in a clinical setting, it may be more beneficial to the patient for the therapy to be implemented in the community (i.e. the patient's home, workplace, gym etc.).

● **Environment:** The environment in which the person lives and functions is important to assess to ensure potential hazards are identified and removed and equipment such as rails are put in place to optimise independence and reduce risk of falling.

● **Balance and vestibular training** Findings from the balance and vestibular assessment should direct which types of interventions are used. For example, if a clinical balance assessment indicates a problem with proprioception and a person with TBI was compensating by fixing their gaze, a range of intervention strategies may be implemented. Altering the surface from a firm to a soft surface, or using a foam mat, will require greater proprioceptive demands. Changing the visual input by asking the person to move their gaze from side to side, or even to close their eyes, will restrict the ability to visually compensate and place greater emphasis on the proprioceptive system. Vestibular dysfunction requires its own particular exercises which are quite distinct from other types of balance exercises.

● **Pain management** Management of a person's pain is not only important to reduce their discomfort and distress, but also to allow rehabilitative efforts to commence. Pain can be a major barrier to engaging in a range of therapies or exercises. Prescription of medication for pain relief before therapy often allows a patient to better engage in therapy, tolerate stretches or tilt-tabling with more comfort and provides greater motivation to move. When a patient reports new or different pain, the relevant investigations are required, as a musculoskeletal injury may have been missed in the acute stage or, alternatively, in the subacute phase, HO may be developing.

● **Maintaining an active lifestyle** All patients, regardless of disability, need to maintain an active lifestyle, with good cardiovascular fitness and body weight. These factors can be very difficult to achieve after TBI, particularly if someone has a dense spastic hemiparesis, which may mean they can only walk indoors with a gait aid. Adaptive equipment such as recumbent bikes, arm ergometers and other machines can be used to achieve a heart rate in a desired training range to meet guidelines for maintaining general health.

This chapter is an abridged version adapted from Williams (2018) with permission.

References

American Congress of Rehabilitation. 1995. Recommendations for use of uniform nomenclature pertinent to patients with severe alterations in consciousness. Archives of Physical Medicine and Rehabilitation 76, 205–209.

Ashworth, B., 1964. Preliminary trial of carisoprodol in multiple sclerosis. Practitioner 192, 540–542.

Berg, K., Wood-Dauphine, S., Williams, J.I., Gayton, D., 1989. Measuring balance in the elderly: preliminary development of an instrument. Physiotherapy Canada 41, 304–311.

Birklein, F., 2005. Complex regional pain syndrome. Journal of Neurology 252, 131–138.

Bohannon, R.W., Smith, M.B., 1987. Interrater reliability of a modified Ashworth scale of muscle spasticity. Physical Therapy 67, 206–207.

Bond, M., 1986. Neurobehavioural sequelae of closed head injury. In: Grant, I., Km, A. (Eds.), Neuropsychological Assessment of Neuropsychiatric Disorders. Oxford University Press, New York.

Bond, R., 1990. Standardised methods for assessing and predicting outcome. In: Rosenthal, M., Griffith, E., Bond, M., Miller, J. (Eds.), Rehabilitation of the Adult and Child with Traumatic Brain Injury. F A Davis, Philadelphia.

Bragge, P., Synnot, A., Maas, A.I., Menon, D.K., Cooper, D.J., Rosenfeld, J.V., Gruen, R.L., 2015. A state-of-the-science overview of randomized controlled trials evaluating acute management of moderate-to-severe traumatic brain injury. Journal of Neurotrauma 33, 1461–1478.

Brashear, A., Elovic, E., 2010. Spasticity: Diagnosis and Management. Demos Medical Publishing, New York.

Bratton, S.L., Chestnut, R.M., Ghajar, J., Mcconnell Hammond, F.F., Harris, O.A., Hartl, R., et al., 2007a. Guidelines for the management of severe traumatic brain injury. II. Hyperosmolar therapy. Journal Neurotrauma. 24 (Suppl. 1), S14–20.

Bratton, S.L., Chestnut, R.M., Ghajar, J., Mcconnell Hammond, F.F., Harris, O.A., Hartl, R., et al., 2007b. Guidelines for the management of severe traumatic brain injury. VIII. Intracranial pressure thresholds. Journal of Neurotrauma. 24 (Suppl. 1), S55–S58.

Brown, R., 2012. Psychological and psychiatric aspects of brain disorder: nature, assessment and implications for clinical neuropsychology. In: Goldstein, L.H., McNeil, J.E. (Eds.), Clinical neuropsychology: a practical guide to assessment and management for clinicians. Wiley Blackwell, Chichester.

Capp, A., Platt, L., 2018. Respiratory management. In: Lennon, S., Ramdharry, G., Verheyden, G. (Eds.), Physical Management for Neurological Conditions. Elsevier Science, London.

Carney, N., Totten, A.M., O'Reilly, C., Ullman, J.S., Hawryluk, G.W.J., Bell, M.J., et al., 2017. Guidelines for the management of severe traumatic brain injury, Fourth Edition. Neurosurgery 80, 6–15.

Crooks, C.Y., Zumsteg, J.M., Bell, K.R., 2007. Traumatic brain injury: a review of practice management and recent advances. Physical Medicine Rehabilitation Clinics North America 18, 681–710, vi.

Daley, K., Mayo, N., Wood-Dauphinee, S., 1999. Reliability of scores on the Stroke Rehabilitation Assessment of Movement (STREAM) measure. Physical Therapy 79, 8–19; quiz 20–23.

de Guise, E., Leblanc, J., Dagher, J., Tinawi, S., Lamoureux, J., Marcoux, J., et al., 2014. Outcome in women with traumatic brain injury admitted to a Level 1 trauma center. International Scholarly Research Notices. https://doi.org/10.1155/2014/263241.

Echemendia, R.J., Meeuwisse, W., Mccrory, P., Davis, G.A., Putukian, M., Leddy, J., et al., 2017. The Sport Concussion Assessment Tool 5th Edition (SCAT5). British Journal of Sports Medicine 51, 851–858.

Flaster, M., Meresh, E., Rao, M., Biller, J., 2013. Central poststroke pain: current diagnosis and treatment. Topics in Stroke Rehabilitation 20, 116–123.

Giacino, J.T., Ashwal, S., Childs, N., Cranford, R., Jennett, B., Katz, D.I., et al., 2002. The minimally conscious state: definition and diagnostic criteria. Neurology. 58, 349–353.

Gorman, S.L., Radtka, S., Melnick, M.E., Abrams, G.M., Byl, N.N., 2010. Development and validation of the function in sitting test in adults with acute stroke. Journal of Neurologic Physical Therapy 34, 150–160.

Haugh, A.B., Pandyan, A.D., Johnson, G.R., 2006. A systematic review of the Tardieu Scale for the measurement of spasticity. Disability and Rehabilitation 28, 899–907.

Ivanhoe, C.B., Reistetter, T.A., 2004. Spasticity: the misunderstood part of the upper motor neuron syndrome. American Journal of Physical Medicine & Rehabilitation 83, S3–S9.

Jennett, B., Snoek, J., Bond, M.R., Brooks, N., 1981. Disability after severe head injury: observations on the Glasgow Coma Scale. Journal of Neurology. Neurosurgery and Psychiatry 44, 285–293.

Jennett, B., Teasdale, G., 1977. Aspects of coma after severe head injury. Lancet. 1, 878–881.

Jeremitsky, E., Omert, L., Dunham, C.M., Protetch, J., Rodriguez, A., 2003. Harbingers of poor outcome the day after severe brain injury: hypothermia, hypoxia, and hypoperfusion. Journal of Trauma 54, 312–319.

Levin, H.S., O'Donnell, V.M., Grossman, R.G., 1979. The Galveston Orientation and Amnesia Test. A Practical Scale to Assess Cognition after Head Injury. Journal of Nervous Mental Disorders 167, 675–684.

Mccrory, P., Meeuwisse, W.H., Aubry, M., Cantu, B., Dvořák, J., Echemendia, R.J., et al., 2013. Consensus statement on concussion in sport: the 4th International Conference on Concussion in Sport held in Zurich, November 2012. British Journal of Sports Medicine 47, 250–258.

Morris, S.L., Dodd, K.J., Morris, M.E., 2004. Outcomes of progressive resistance strength training following stroke: a systematic review. Clinical Rehabilitation 18, 27–39.

New Zealand Guidelines Group, 2006. Traumatic brain injury: diagnosis, acute management and rehabilitation [Online]. Wellington, New Zealand: New Zealand Guidelines Group. Available at: http://www.moh.govt.nz/NoteBook/nbbooks.nsf/0/B8738C36058 89A6ACC257A6D00809243? [Accessed 15.05.2018.].

O'Connor, P., 2002. Hospitalisation due to traumatic brain injury (TBI), Australia 1997-98. Adelaide: Australian Institute of Health and Welfare.

O'Connor, P.J., Cripps, R.A., 1999. Traumatic brain injury (TBI) surveillance issues. Adelaide: AIHW National Injury Surveillance Unit, Flinders University Research Centre for Injury Studies.

Olver, J., Esquenazi, A., Fung, V., Singer, B., Ward, A., 2010. Botulinum toxin assessment, intervention and aftercare for lower limb disorders of movement and muscle tone in adults: international consensus statement. European Journal of Neurology 17, 57–73.

Perrin, P.B., Niemeier, J.P., Mougeot, J.-L., Vannoy, C.H., Hirsch, M.A., Watts, J.A., et al., 2015. Measures of injury severity and prediction of acute traumatic brain injury outcomes. The Journal of head trauma rehabilitation 30, 136–42.

Ponsford, J., 2014. Lomgitudinal follow-up of patients with traumatic brain injury: outcome at two, five and ten years. Journal of Neurotrauma. 31, 64–77.

Ponsford, J., Sloan, S., Snow, P., 2013. Traumatic brain injury: rehabilitation for everyday adaptive living. Psychology Press East Sussex.

Ponsford, J.L., Olver, J.H., Curran, C., 1995. A profile of outcome: 2 years after traumatic brain injury. Brain Injury 9, 1–10.

Schonberger, M., Ponsford, J., Olver, J., Ponsford, M., Wirtz, M., 2011. Prediction of functional and employment outcome 1 year after traumatic brain injury: a structural equation modelling approach. Journal of Neurology, Neurosurgery, and Psychiatry 82, 936–941.

Scottish Intercollegiate Guidelines Network (SIGN), 2013. Brain injury rehabilitation in adults. A national clinical guideline. Scottish Intercollegiate Guidelines Network (SIGN), Edinburgh.

Seel, R.T., Sherer, M., Whyte, J., Katz, D.I., Giacino, J.T., Rosenbaum, A.M., et al., 2010. Assessment scales for disorders of consciousness: evidence-based recommendations for clinical practice and research. Archives of Physical Medicine and Rehabilitation 91, 1795–1813.

Sheean, G., Lannin, N., Turner-Stokes, L., Rawicki, B., Snow, B., 2010. Botulinum toxin assessment, intervention and after-care for upper limb hypertonicity in adults: international consensus statement. European Journal of Neurology 17, 74–93.

Shores, E.A., Marosszeky, J.E., Sandanam, J., Batchelor, J., 1986. Preliminary validation of a clinical scale for measuring the duration of post-traumatic amnesia. Medical Journal of Australia 144, 569–572.

Singer, B.J., Jegasothy, G.M., Singer, K.P., Allison, G.T., 2003. Evaluation of serial casting to correct equinovarus deformity of the ankle after acquired brain injury in adults. Archives of Physical Medicine and Rehabilitation 84, 483–491.

Stark, T., Walker, B., Phillips, J.K., Fejer, R., Beck, R., 2011. Hand-held dynamometry correlation with the gold standard isokinetic dynamometry: a systematic review. Physical Medicine and Rehabilitation 3, 472–479.

State of Colorado, 2013. Traumatic brain injury medical treatment guidelines. In: Department of Labor and Employment, D. O. W. C, fourth ed. Colorado, USA: State of Colorado.

Sullivan, K.J., Cen, S.Y., 2011. Model of disablement and recovery: knowledge translation in rehabilitation research and practice. Physical Therapy 91, 1892–1904.

Taylor, N.F., Dodd, K.J., Damiano, D.L., 2005. Progressive resistance exercise in physical therapy: a summary of systematic reviews. Physical Therapy 85, 1208–1223.

Teasdale, G., Jennett, B., 1974. Assessment of coma and impaired consciousness. A practical scale. Lancet. 2, 81–84.

Turner-Stokes, L.F., Williams, H., Bill, A., Bassett, P., Sephton, K., 2016. Cost-efficiency of inpatient specialist rehabilitation following acquired brain injury: a large multi-centre cohort analysis from the UK. Brain Injury. https://doi.org/10.1136/bmjopen-2015-010238.

Verplancke, D., Snape, S., Salisbury, C.F., Jones, P.W., Ward, A.B., 2005. A randomized controlled trial of botulinum toxin on lower limb spasticity following acute acquired severe brain injury. Clinical Rehabilitation 19, 117–125.

Williams, G., Kahn, M., Randall, A., 2014. Strength training for walking in neurologic rehabilitation is not task specific: a focused review. American Journal of Physical Medicine & Rehabilitation 93, 511–522.

Williams, G., 2018. Traumatic brain injury. In: Lennon, S., Ramdharry, G., Verheyden, G. (Eds.), Physical Management for Neurological Conditions. Elsevier Science, London.

Wilson, C., 2018. Clinical neuropsychology. In: Lennon, S., Ramdharry, G., Verheyden, G. (Eds.), Physical Management for Neurological Conditions. Elsevier Science, London.

CHAPTER 10

Spinal cord injury

Sue Paddison and Benita Hexter

INTRODUCTION

Spinal cord injury (SCI) denotes disruption of the neural tissue within the spinal canal. It refers to damage to the cord resulting from trauma, disease or degeneration, which presents as an upper motor neurone lesion with varying loss of sensation, weakness and spasticity. Vertebral injury below T12 will often result in cauda equina syndrome (CES) as the spinal cord ends at the L1 or L2 vertebral level. There may also be intracanal damage to the brachial plexus or other peripheral nerves. These injuries result in a lower motor neurone lesion which is characterised by the absence of spasticity. Paraplegia is used to describe dysfunction of the trunk and lower limbs arising from damage to the spinal cord below T1. Tetraplegia refers to loss of function in the upper limbs, trunk and lower limbs caused by injury at cervical spinal levels. See special considerations for children available at www.spinalcordinjury.nhs.uk. The management of SCI is complex (NHS England Service Standards 2014). Although the most obvious impairments are paralysis and sensory loss, SCI affects many other body functions, including cardiovascular, bowel and bladder, respiratory, gastrointestinal and sexual function.

EPIDEMIOLOGY

- Estimated to be around 40–80 cases per million population (www.WHO.int 2013, Wyndaele & Wyndaele 2006).
- The ratio of male to female cases is approximately 2:1, with greater male preponderance in young age groups.
- SCI in children is rare and mostly results from trauma.
- Spinal cord damage can be traumatic or nontraumatic.

INCIDENCE

- Approximately 1200 people in the UK are paralysed from SCI per year – one every 8 hours.
- An estimated 8 people/million experience a nontraumatic injury.

AETIOLOGY

- Traumatic injuries may lead to vascular and compressive damage with bony and/or ligamentous disruption.
- Nontraumatic aetiology is caused by ischaemic damage (spinal stroke; ruptured aortic aneurysm or arteriovenous malformation), degenerative disc disease, spinal canal stenosis, viral and bacterial infective diseases (transverse myelitis), tumours or abscesses (often tuberculous).
- There are more incomplete than complete lesions.
- There are an increasing number of older people with SCI largely caused by falls.

PATHOPHYSIOLOGY

Most traumatic injuries involve contusion or tearing of the underlying cord by displaced bony fragments, disc or ligaments. Secondary damage results from swelling and increasing cord pressure affecting the venous and arterial supply and results in ischaemia, lack of necessary proteins and failure to remove the debris of injury. Neurological recovery is further hindered by the inflammatory processes.

DIAGNOSIS

- Based on the International Standard Neurological Classification of Spinal Cord Injury (ISNCSCI) still commonly referred to as the *ASIA test* (American Spinal Injuries Association) (Fig. 10.1). Online training is freely available at www.asia-spinalinjury.org/learning.
- The level represents the highest (most cephalad) myotome and dermatome in which normal function is preserved and describes how much function is maintained below the level of injury, ranging from A (no function to S4 and S5) to E (normal function).

PROGNOSIS

- Ninety per cent of incomplete tetraplegics (Asia Impairment Scale (AIS) C and D) SCI patients have some recovery of a motor level in their upper limbs compared with 70% to 85% of the complete injuries (AIS A and B) (Ditunno et al 2000).
- Pinprick preservation below the level of the injury to the sacral dermatomes is the best indicator of useful recovery, with 75% of patients regaining the ability to walk (van Middendorp et al 2011).
- Functional outlines are presented in Table 10.1.

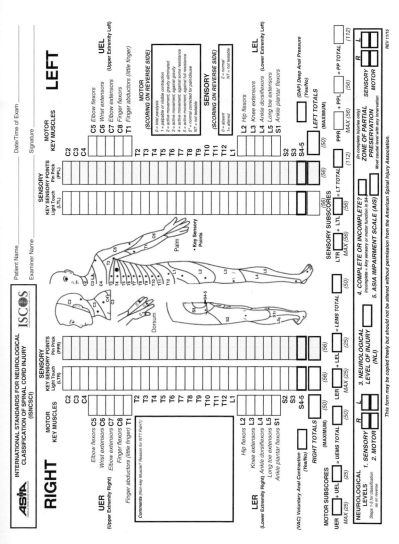

Fig. 10.1
International Standard Neurological Classification of Spinal Cord Injury worksheet.

Muscle Function Grading

0 = total paralysis

1 = palpable or visible contraction

2 = active movement, full range of motion (ROM) with gravity eliminated

3 = active movement, full ROM against gravity

4 = active movement, full ROM against gravity and moderate resistance in a muscle specific position

5 = (normal) active movement, full ROM against gravity and full resistance in a functional muscle position expected from an otherwise unimpaired person

5* = (normal) active movement, full ROM against gravity and sufficient resistance to be considered normal if identified inhibiting factors (i.e. pain, disuse) were not present

NT = not testable (i.e. due to immobilization, severe pain such that the patient cannot be graded, amputation of limb, or contracture of > 50% of the normal ROM)

Sensory Grading

0 = Absent

1 = Altered, either decreased/impaired sensation or hypersensitivity

2 = Normal

NT = Not testable

When to Test Non-Key Muscles:

In a patient with an apparent AIS B classification, non-key muscle functions more than 3 levels below the motor level on each side should be tested to most accurately classify the injury (differentiate between AIS B and C).

Movement	Root level
Shoulder: Flexion, extension, abduction, adduction, internal and external rotation **Elbow:** Supination	C5
Elbow: Pronation **Wrist:** Flexion	C6
Finger: Flexion at proximal joint, extension. **Thumb:** Flexion, extension and abduction in plane of thumb	C7
Finger: Flexion at MCP joint **Thumb:** Opposition, adduction and abduction perpendicular to palm	C8
Finger: Abduction of the index finger	T1
Hip: Adduction	L2
Hip: External rotation	L3
Hip: Extension, abduction, internal rotation **Knee:** Flexion **Ankle:** Inversion and eversion **Toe:** MP and IP extension	L4
Hallux and Toe: DIP and PIP flexion and abduction	L5
Hallux: Adduction	S1

ASIA Impairment Scale (AIS)

A = Complete. No sensory or motor function is preserved in the sacral segments S4-5.

B = Sensory Incomplete. Sensory but not motor function is preserved below the neurological level and includes the sacral segments S4-5 (light touch or pin prick at S4-5 or deep anal pressure) AND no motor function is preserved more than three levels below the motor level on either side of the body.

C = Motor Incomplete. Motor function is preserved at the most caudal sacral segments for voluntary anal contraction (VAC) OR the patient meets the criteria for sensory incomplete status (sensory function preserved at the most caudal sacral segments (S4-S5) by LT, PP or DAP), and has some sparing of motor function more than three levels below the ipsilateral motor level on either side of the body. (This includes key or non-key muscle functions to determine motor incomplete status.) For AIS C – less than half of key muscle functions below the single NLI have a muscle grade ≥ 3.

D = Motor Incomplete. Motor incomplete status as defined above, with at least half (half or more) of key muscle functions below the single NLI having a muscle grade ≥ 3.

E = Normal. If sensation and motor function as tested with the ISNCSCI are graded as normal in all segments, and the patient had prior deficits, then the AIS grade is E. Someone without an initial SCI does not receive an AIS grade.

Using ND: To document the sensory, motor and NLI levels, the ASIA Impairment Scale grade, and/or the zone of partial preservation (ZPP) when they are unable to be determined based on the examination results.

Steps in Classification

The following order is recommended for determining the classification of individuals with SCI.

1. Determine sensory levels for right and left sides.
The sensory level is the most caudal, intact dermatome for both pin prick and light touch sensation.

2. Determine motor levels for right and left sides.
Defined by the lowest key muscle function that has a grade of at least 3 (on supine testing), providing the key muscle functions represented by segments above that level are judged to be intact (graded as a 5).
Note: in regions where there is no myotome to test, the motor level is presumed to be the same as the sensory level, if testable motor function above that level is also normal.

3. Determine the neurological level of injury (NLI)
This refers to the most caudal segment of the cord with intact sensation and antigravity (3 or more) muscle function strength, provided that there is normal (intact) sensory and motor function rostrally respectively.
The NLI is the most cephalad of the sensory and motor levels determined in steps 1 and 2.

4. Determine whether the injury is Complete or Incomplete.
(i.e. absence or presence of sacral sparing)
If voluntary anal contraction = **No** AND all S4-5 sensory scores = **0** AND deep anal pressure = **No**, then injury is **Complete.**
Otherwise, injury is **Incomplete.**

5. Determine ASIA Impairment Scale (AIS) Grade:

Is injury Complete? If YES, AIS=A and can record ZPP (lowest dermatome or myotome on each side with some preservation)

NO ↓

Is injury Motor Complete? If YES, AIS=B
(No = voluntary anal contraction OR motor function more than three levels below the motor level on a given side, if the patient has sensory incomplete classification)

NO ↓

Are at least half (half or more) of the key muscles below the neurological level of injury graded 3 or better?

NO → AIS=C   YES → AIS=D

If sensation and motor function is normal in all segments, AIS=E

Note: AIS E is used in follow-up testing when an individual with a documented SCI has recovered normal function. If at initial testing no deficits are found, the individual is neurologically intact; the ASIA Impairment Scale does not apply.

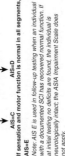

INTERNATIONAL STANDARDS FOR NEUROLOGICAL CLASSIFICATION OF SPINAL CORD INJURY

AMERICAN SPINAL INJURY ASSOCIATION

ISCOS
INTERNATIONAL SPINAL CORD SOCIETY

Fig. 10.1, cont'd.

Table 10.1 Functional outcomes after spinal cord injury

Level of complete spinal cord injury and key movements added at that level	Maximal functional potential
C0–C4 24 hr ventilated head and neck flexion and rotation, scapula elevation	Verbally independent in postural adjustment
	Acceptable posture and seating and skin integrity equipment provided
	Head/chin control–powered wheelchair
	Potential use of assistive technology for communication and environmental control
	Verbally independent in directing own care
	Able to stand using device with assistance
C0–C4 night ventilated	Inspiratory muscle training programme
C0–C4 not ventilated	Up in wheelchair for 12 consecutive hours
C5 biceps rotator cuff shoulder abduction	Upper limb–controlled powered mobility
	Self-propelling wheelchair
	Assisted same height transfer on and off bed with aids (not including lifting legs)
	Once set up with adaptive aids, carry out grooming activities in an accessible environment
	Once with set up with adaptive aids, carry out feeding in an accessible environment
	Once set up with adaptive aids, carry out writing in an accessible environment
C6 wrist extension	Independent pressure relief
	Independent positioning in Wheelchair
	Self-propelling on level surfaces
	Self-propelling on small inclines
	Independent flipping front castors
	Independent back wheel balance
	Independent traversing of rough terrain in back-wheel balance
	Independent ascending and descending 7.5-cm kerb
	Independent rolling in double bed
	Independent moving between supine lying and long sitting in bed

(continued)

Table 10.1 Functional outcomes after spinal cord injury—cont'd

Level of complete spinal cord injury and key movements added at that level	Maximal functional potential
	Independent lifting of legs on and off the bed
	Independent same-height transfers with transfer board (TB) on and off bed
	Assisted car transfers with TB
	Independent lifting of lightweight wheelchair in and out of car
	Independent grooming in an accessible environment
	Independent writing in an accessible environment
	Independent feeding in an accessible environment
	Independent light daily activities of daily living (DADLs)
	Independent in upper limb personal activities of daily living (PADL) with adaptive aids
	Independent in lower limb PADL with adaptive aids
C7 elbow extension	Possibility of supported ambulation options
	Independent car transfers with TB
	Independent graduated floor to w/c transfer
	Independent same-height transfers on/off bed with no aids
	Independent stretch programme
C8/T1 finger and thumb movement	Independent in upper limb PADL without aids in an accessible environment
	Independent in lower limb PADL without aids in an accessible environment
	Independent in light DADL without aids in an accessible environment
	Independent in/out standing frame
T2–T6 increasing trunk stabilisers	Upstairs/downstairs in wheelchair with assistance
	'Bunny hop' in wheelchair
	Independent floor to and from wheelchair transfer
	Independent car transfers with no aids
	Independent in heavy DADL without aids in an accessible environment
T7–T12 abdominals	Potential for ambulation with KAFO
L1–L2 hip flexion	Consideration of functional ambulation

Table 10.1 Functional outcomes after spinal cord injury—cont'd

Level of complete spinal cord injury and key movements added at that level	Maximal functional potential
L3 knee extension	Independent indoor functional ambulation
L4–L5 dorsiflexion S1–S5 plantarflexion knee flexion hip extension	Independent ascend/descend 7.5-cm step/kerb with no rail
	Independent ascend/descend flight of stairs
	Independent on/off floor
	Independent ascend/descend 1:12 slope
	Independent outdoor functional ambulation

From SCIFERTO Spinal Cord Injury Therapy Leads 2016.
C0 no level of normal spinal cord function preserved.

INCOMPLETE SYNDROMES

There are recognised patterns of incomplete cord injury where the signs and symptoms are related to the anatomical areas of the cord affected. Clinically, patterns of incomplete lesions are referred to as a syndrome (Kirshblum et al 2011). The most common syndromes are presented in Table 10.2.

Table 10.2 Common patterns of incomplete lesions

Syndrome	Frequency	Location	Common mechanism	Consequences	Prognosis
Anterior cord syndrome	44%	Anterior two thirds of spinal cord or anterior spinal artery	High-velocity hyperflexion	Reduced motor function Reduced sensation to pain and temperature Proprioception preserved	Poor 10%–20% potential of motor recovery (Sheerin 2005)
Cauda equina syndrome	25%	Compression of the sacral nerve roots	Intervertebral disc herniation	Flaccid paralysis caused by peripheral nerve damage Flaccid paralysis of bowel and bladder	Rate of residual dysfunction: Micturition 38%, defecation 43% and sexual dysfunction 54% (Korse et al 2017)

(continued)

Table 10.2 Common patterns of incomplete lesions—cont'd

Syndrome	Frequency	Location	Common mechanism	Consequences	Prognosis
Brown–Séquard syndrome	17%	Hemisection of spinal cord	Shot or stab wound	Greater ipsilateral proprioceptive and motor loss Contralateral loss of sensitivity to pain and temperature	75%–90% of individuals ambulate postrehabilitation (Johnston 2001)
Central cord syndrome	10%	Compression injury Degenerative changes in the spinal column Osteophytes Disc bulges Spondylitic joint Hyperextension injuries	Often after a fall in the older population	Upper limbs are more affected than the lower limbs Some flaccid weakness of the arms resulting from lower motor neurone lesions at the level of injury Partial bowel and bladder dysfunctions	57%–86% patients will ambulate, although 97% of younger patients less than 50 years ambulate compared with 41% over 50 years (Foo 1986)

From McKinley et al 2007.

EARLY ACUTE MANAGEMENT

- Surgical decompression and stabilisation may be necessary, or conservative treatment regimens may be followed with bed rest, careful rolling and positioning, possibly supplemented with traction (MASCIP Turning Guidelines 2015) and orthotic devices (see precautions in Box 10.1).
- Orthostatic changes in blood pressure can be problematic on initial mobilisation, requiring careful management of blood pressure (Alexander et al 2009). Use of physical compression may limit symptoms, such as T.E.D. stockings and elastic abdominal binders.
- The main objectives in the acute phase are to (Johnston 2001):
    - institute a prophylactic respiratory regimen and treat any complications;
    - achieve independent respiratory status where possible;
    - maintain full range of motion (ROM) of all joints within the limitations determined by fracture stability (see precautions in Box 10.1);
    - monitor and manage neurological status as appropriate;
    - maintain/strengthen all innervated muscle groups;

- facilitate functional patterns of activity to assist in restoration of function where possible;
- support/educate the patient, carers, family and colleagues.

Box 10.1 Precautions with unstable spinal cord injury

1. Undertake facilitated movements in supine position.
2. Unstable paraplegic spinal cord injury (SCI) (T9 and below):
   - Limit hip flexion to 30 degrees (tailor position for knee flexion).
3. Unstable tetraplegic SCI (T4 level and above):
   - Shoulder hold during lower limb movements and upper limb movements above 90 degrees.
4. Severe spasms during limb movements may cause loss of spinal alignment:
   - Use shoulder hold.
5. Respiratory techniques should be applied bilaterally with a shoulder hold.
6. Extreme range of movement must be avoided.

RESPIRATORY MANAGEMENT (SEE ALSO CHAPTER 7)

- SCI can result in paralysis of respiratory muscles of inspiration (diaphragm to C5 and intercostals to corresponding thoracic level) and muscles of expiration (abdominals: T6–T12). The patient's cough will be impaired to varying degrees if the level of the lesion is T12 or above. Cough will be significantly impaired above level T6. See assessment in Tables 10.3 & 10.4.
- An unstable spinal column may preclude use of manual techniques or require them to be done in supine position with a shoulder hold where necessary (see Box 10.2).
- Because of the autonomic changes, there is a high risk of cardiac instability. Bradycardia resulting from unopposed vagal stimulation is common and can be exacerbated by tracheal suction.
- If forced vital capacity (FVC) descends below 500 mL, some invasive or non-invasive ventilator support will be required. If FVC drops below 1 litre, positive pressure respiratory support is recommended (RISCI Guidelines 2010).
- Critical values for peak expiratory flow rate (PEFR):
  - <280 L/min: cough may not be effective
  - <160 L/min: ineffective cough
- There is some evidence of positive effect of inspiratory muscle training on lung volumes, respiratory muscle strength and perception of dyspnoea (Berlowitz & Tamplin 2013).

Box 10.2 Precautions in the use of respiratory techniques

Unstable spinal column:
- Treat in supine position
- Bilateral chest techniques with shoulder hold
- Caution with manual assisted cough with shoulder hold

Manual assisted cough:
- The aim is to replace the compressive effect of the abdominal musculature using the hands or forearm of an assistant, timed with a deep breath and an active cough.
- Contraindicated if there is a paralytic ileus, severe constipation or abdominal injuries.
- Use caution with chest or abdominal injuries and pathologies, clotting disorders, unstable angina and cardiac arrhythmias.

Suction:
- Undertake suction with care.
- During suction the vagus nerve is unopposed and the patient may become hypotensive and bradycardiac, possibly resulting in cardiac arrest.

Table 10.3 Respiratory assessment

Subjective assessment		Objective assessment
Level of spinal cord injury		Respiratory rate
Spinal precautions		SaO_2
Other injuries		FiO_2
Cardiac stability		Heart rate
Past medical history (PMH) – Chronic obstructive pulmonary disease (COPD), asthma, smoking		Blood pressure
Age		Fluid balance
Cardiovascular fitness		Temperature
Drug history (DH)	steroids	Auscultation
	anticoagulants	Cough
	inotropes for cardiac contractility	Breathing pattern
Bowel management		Abdomen
Ventilation method and history		Forced vital capacity
		Cough peak expiratory flow rate
		Chest x-ray
		ABGs

From McKinley et al 2007.

Table 10.4 Forced vital capacity (FVC) values in spinal cord injury

	FVC % normal predicted motor completes	FVC % normal predicted motor incompletes
C3	52	58
C7	67	84
T6	84	99
L1	95	96

From Linn et al 2001.

Weaning from Ventilatory Support (RISCI Weaning Guidelines 2017)

- Prerequisites for the initiation of weaning are:
  - FiO_2 <0.4;
  - PEEP preferably around 5 cm H_2O;
  - awake and cooperative;
- minimal opiates;
  - no active sepsis;
  - some evidence of spontaneous respiratory activity.

Long-Term Respiratory Management

- Ongoing use of incentive spirometry and muscle training devices is potentially beneficial for all those with significant respiratory deficit.
- Teaching of a self manual assisted cough (MAC) for those who are able and training care staff in MAC is essential for those with impaired coughs.
- In the long term, those with a large degree of impairment to coughs may benefit from a domestic cough assist device.
- For some, ongoing use of noninvasive or mandatory ventilation may be required.

CLINICAL PRESENTATION

Acute traumatic management guidelines are well established (NICE 2016). The function of all systems below the level of lesion will be changed. Comprehensive multidisciplinary guidelines in SCI management are also widely available (ISCoS 2015). Key points are:

- Spinal shock: The transient suppression and gradual return of reflex activity below the cord lesion (Dittuno et al 2004).
- Weakness: Some muscles may be completely denervated, whereas others retain partial innervation.
- Sensory changes: Absence of sensation occurs; parasthaesia is common.
- Balance dysfunction.
- Spasticity: Affects about 65%, with 35% needing treatment for clonus and spasms (Holtz et al 2017).

10

- Autonomic dysfunction: There is altered control of the bowel and bladder, blood vessels, the heart and lungs and all organs (Tator 1998).
- Cardiovascular dysfunction: Injury at or above T1–T5 will interrupt sympathetic activity. The unopposed parasympathetic stimulation results in persistent bradycardia.
- Hypotension resulting in dizziness and fainting. Supportive abdominal elasticated binders and compression stockings are routinely used to support blood pressure.
- Thermoregulation: Altered control of smooth muscle may lead to poikilothermia and limbs feeling cold and discolouring (Schubert & Fagrell 1991).
- Autonomic dysreflexia (AD): an exaggerated sympathetic nervous system response in lesions above T6 to noxious stimuli below the level of spinal cord injury. Consequent hypertension may become a medical emergency and if untreated, result in stroke and death. AD effects 50-70% of those with cervical injuries (Karlsson, 2006). It can result in hypertension, bradycardia and headache with piloerection and capillary dilation and sweating, above the level of the lesion. The sudden absence of higher control of sympathetic function above T6 results in neurogenic shock, characterised by bradycardia and low blood pressure (Table 10.5).
- Bladder dysfunction: Incomplete emptying may increase risk of bladder infections and damage the urinary and renal system because of high pressures as urine accumulates.
- Bowel dysfunction: Changes in the peristaltic activity of the bowel and paralysis of the anal sphincter result in constipation and continence issues. Training the bowel habit for UMN lesions can restore continence with a degree of reliability (MASCIP Bowel Guidelines 2012).

Table 10.5 Key factors in autonomic dysreflexia

Signs and symptoms	Potential causes	Responses required
• Increased blood pressure (>20% increase in systolic blood pressure above baseline) (Alexander et al 2009) • Rash above level of injury • Pounding headache • Goose bumps above level of spinal cord injury • Bradycardia or tachycardia • Nasal congestion • Vascular constriction below level of injury	• Severe spasticity • Sudden stretch • Fractures • Skin breakdown • Ingrown toenail • Sepsis (particularly bladder) • Full bladder (blocked catheter) • Constipation.	• Sit patient upright • Loosen clothing • Check for and manage any cause of bladder or bowel irritation • Check for and manage other potential triggers • Consider pharmacological management if unable to identify and remove the trigger

- Sexual dysfunction: Erectile dysfunction is a common consequence. Reflex erection often occurs in UMN lesions. Fertility is not impaired in women; men often require in vitro fertilisation (IVF) to become fathers.
- Pain: Affects 40% to 50% of SCI patients (Brix Finnerup 2013). A lack of sensation or movement in a part of the body does not mean that pain cannot be experienced there. Neuropathic pain results from sensitisation of input into the dorsal horn and to the damaged neural structures (Nepomuceno et al 1979).

ASSESSMENT

Subjective assessment is presented in Table 10.6. Objectively, it is essential to assess weakness, sensation, spasticity/tone, range of motion, and the impact of these impairments at the level of activity and participation. Consideration should be given to technique, assistance, aids and appliances in the performance of transfers, bed mobility and ambulation. Common outcome measures are presented in Table 10.7.

Table 10.6 Subjective assessment

HPC:	• date of SCI • mode of SCI • skeletal spinal Injury • other injuries at time of SCI • spinal surgery	• other surgery • inpatient rehabilitation • outpatient/community rehabilitation • current ISNCSCI
DH:	• anticoagulants • steroids • Botulinum toxin	• antispasmodics • pain medication
PMH:	• osteoporosis/osteopenia • heterotrophic ossification • rheumatoid arthritis • fractures (other than at time of SCI) • musculoskeletal injuries • hypertension • cardiovascular disease • diabetes	• surgery • COPD • DVT/PE • malignancy • autonomic dysreflexia • pacemakers/implants • psychological wellbeing
SH:	• home • house/flat • permanent/temporary • owned/privately rented/HA/council • steps and stairs inside • steps and stairs to access • bedroom	• bathrooms • others in residence • home roles and responsibilities • work • driving/transport • leisure/hobbies/interests • care

(continued)

Table 10.6 Subjective assessment—cont'd

| Currently: | ● spasticity/spasms
● pain
● skin
● bowel/bladder
● exercise programme
● respiratory
● fitness activities
● standing | ● mobility – indoor, outdoor, important environments
● orthotics
● wheelchair/posture/seating
● ADLs/function
● weight
● sleeping
● mood |

HPC, History of presenting complaint; *ISNCSCI,* International Standard Neurological Classification of Spinal Cord Injury; *DH,* drug history; *PMH,* past medical history; *COPD,* chronic obstructive pulmonary disease; *DVT,* deep venous thrombosis; *PE,* pulmonary embolism; *HA,* housing authority; *ADL,* activities of daily living.

Table 10.7 Common outcome measures in spinal cord injury

Fitness	Borg Perceived Rate of Exertion				
	(Borg 1982)				
Gait	WISCI II	10-metre walk	6-minute walk	Berg Balance Scale	SCI FAI
	(Ditunno et al, 2008, Ditunno & Ditunno 2001)	(Amatachaya et al 2014)		(Berg 1993)	(Field-Fote 2001)
ODFS	PCI				
	(MacGregor 1981)				
Respiratory	Cough PEFR	FVC			
SCI	ISNCSCI	SCIM III		Chart	
		(Catz et al 2007)		(Whiteneck et al 1992)	
Spasticity	Modified Ashworth Scale		Penn Spasm Frequency Scale		ROM
	(Bohannon & Smith 1987)		(Penn et al 1989)		
Upper Limbs	Wheelchair User's Shoulder Pain Index (WUSPI)				
	(Curtis et al 1995)				

WISCI II, Walking index for spinal cord injury; *SCI,* Spinal cord injury; *FAI,* Functional ambulation inventory; *ODFS,* Odstock drop foot stimulator; *PCI,* Physiological cost index; *PEFR,* Peak expiratory flow rate; *FVC,* Forced vital capacity; *ISNCSCI:* International standard neurological classification of spinal cord Injury; *SCIM,* Spinal cord independence measure; *ROM,* Range of movement; *WUSPI,* Wheelchair user's shoulder Pain index.

REHABILITATION

Guidance for rehabilitation goals and techniques can be found at:

● www.elearnsci.org. Further reading on physiotherapy in SCI can be found in Harvey et al (2016a; 2016b).

The aims of rehabilitation are to:

- establish an interdisciplinary process that is patient focused, comprehensive and coordinated;
- address physical needs with early intervention and prophylaxis to prevent further complications;
- deliver information to equip the individual with knowledge to achieve independence;
- gain independence, whether physical or verbal, and equipment provision to facilitate this independence;
- achieve and maintain successful reintegration into the community and vocation;
- manage psychological adaptation to the newly acquired physical condition.

Therapists focus on the following interventions during the rehabilitation phase:

- Respiratory care
- Maintaining ROM and preventing contracture
  - Take joints and muscles through their full available range on a daily basis. The effectiveness of stretch and passive movements is controversial (Harvey et al 2017).
  - Use positioning to avoid adoption of potentially problematic postures and protect end of range of vulnerable joints (Box 10.3).

Box 10.3 Recommendations for positioning in bed

- Cervical spine in neutral (avoidance of prolonged flexion)
- Elbow extension in pronation and supination
- Shoulder abduction and external rotation
- Prone lying
- Alternating between hip and knee flexion and extension
- Dorsiflexion
- 'Frogged' position – supine with hips flexed and externally rotated, knees flexed

- Splinting may be necessary to maintain ROM, particularly when unopposed activity and significant spasticity are present (ACPIN 2014; see Box 10.4).

Box 10.4 Reasons to consider splinting (ACPIN 2014)

- Reduce oedema
- Maintain soft tissue length
- Prevent overstretching

Continued

Box 10.4 Reasons to consider splinting (ACPIN 2014)—cont'd

- Support anatomical alignment
- Prevent contractures and deformity with prolonged stretch
- Manage spasticity
- Promote function
- Replace function

- Strength training: Consider facilitated, gravity eliminated, gravity opposed to resisted exercises, and hydrotherapy (Box 10.5).

Box 10.5 Strength training principles in spinal cord injury (Bye et al 2017)

In fully innervated muscles:
- Hypertrophy:
    4 × 10 repetitions, 20 isometric, 20 concentric to exhaustion at end of each set of 10
For partially innervated muscles:
- Neuromuscular electrical stimulation in upper motor neurone lesion (with an intact peripheral nerve supply)
- Direct muscle stimulation in lower motor neurone injury

- Balance training: Sitting supported in the wheelchair is progressed to sitting on a plinth with bilateral arm support to unilateral to no arm support incorporating reaching activities.
- Implementing a daily standing programme:
    - The use of devices (tilt table, standing frames) to support a standing position two to three times per week for up to 1 hour is recommended for everyone (MASCIP Standing Guidelines 2013).
- Functional mobility:
    - Rolling side to side using upper limbs to gain momentum; prone; lying to sitting; long sitting for hamstring stretching, balance and push ups (see Bromley 2006).
    - Some movements that are absent can be retrained in a different way using substitute movements (Mateo et al 2015). For example, tenodesis is a functional grip for C6/C7 injuries that utilises activity in wrist extensors to bring about passive opposition of the thumb and finger flexion to grip and to release when the wrist is flexed (Fig. 10.2). When facilitating a tenodesis grip, passive movements in wrist neutral should include wrist extension with finger flexion and wrist flexion with finger extension.
    - Transfers: Lifting in preparation for transfer begins on the plinth initially with hand blocks. A transfer board may be used for legs-up and legs-down

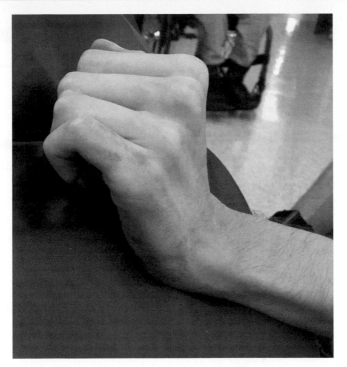

Fig. 10.2
Tenodesis Grip.

transfers on to the bed. More challenging transfers require practice in lifting from various levels for functional activities: between two plinths; floor to plinth; floor to chair; chair to car, bath and easy chair.

- Wheelchair prescription and seating: Careful choice of cushion and chair is required. Teaching hourly forward leaning pressure relief, chest on lap, arms dangling forward, for 2 consecutive minutes found to be the optimum for allowing capillary reperfusion. Those who cannot should be able to instruct those assisting them. Essential principles of safety and wheelchair skills are taught (varied height kerbs, slopes, uneven terrain, tight corners and, if possible, stairs and escalator techniques). (See Table 10.8).

- Gait training: Technological advances such as treadmill training with body weight support, robotics and exoskeletons are challenging to implement because of high costs and accessibility for the majority of people with SCI (Boninger et al 2012). They can be used to supplement therapeutic handling in the fulfilment of the potential for ambulation.

Table 10.8 Checklist for good seated posture

Body segment	Optimal position
Trunk	● Adequate lumbar lordosis supported by a back rest ● Buttocks back in the chair
Pelvis	● Neutral position ● Avoid posterior tilt ● Neutral lateral alignment (indicated by level ASIS [Anterior Superior Anterior Spine])
Arms	● Arms should rest without scapula elevation but high enough to reduce any glenohumeral subluxation ● Able to reach, when possible, without stabilising with other arm or falling forward
Thighs	● Thighs supported on cushion, which should finish 2–3 cm behind the knees ● Hips in neutral rotation, using inserts if required
Knees	● 90 degrees flexion and aligned over ankles
Ankle	● Plantargrade, with soles of feet well supported

● Walking orthoses, including knee ankle foot orthoses (KAFOs), may be used to optimise gait and support walking in those with a complete paraplegia. Criteria to consider before calliper training:
  ● sufficient upper-limb strength to lift body weight;
  ● no upper limb injuries;
  ● full ROM of hips, knees and ankles;
  ● cardiovascular fitness sufficient to sustain walking activity;
  ● assessment of spinal deformity (e.g. scoliosis) that may hinder standing balance;
  ● motivation of the patient;
  ● assessment of spasticity that may make walking unsafe.
● Fitness training: Consider group exercise, sport and circuit training and functional electrical stimulation (FES) ergometry (Ptasinski 2010).
  ● Recommendation: Twenty minutes of moderate to vigorous intensity exercise, two times a week, and strength training exercises two times a week, consisting of three sets of 8 to 10 repetitions of each exercise for each major muscle group (SCI Action Canada 2011).

Special considerations

● Reduced bone density: There is an increased risk of fractures associated with osteopenia and osteoporosis, with some evidence to suggest a passive standing programme and FES ergometry can reduce demineralisation in some bones (Soleyman-Jahi et al 2017).

- Shoulder pain: Careful positioning in the acute phase can prevent early problems from developing. Additional support from Lycra garments across the shoulder may provide relief for those with limited arm function.
  - Enhancing stability through adequate seating may help avoid impingement.
  - Specific exercises to address muscle imbalance and maintenance of full range of motion have been shown to reduce incidence of pain (van Straaten et al 2017).
  - Options for reducing strain on the upper limbs should be considered, with good transfer technique, appropriate environments, minimising the need for overhead reaching and the use of power-assisted wheelchair options being a starting point.
- Tissue viability: Sensation is impaired. Tissues are less able to tolerate compression and heal less efficiently because of reduction in circulation and reduced muscle activity. Reduced muscle mass often leaves bony prominences more exposed.
  - Implementation of a regular turning regimen should be developed to reduce pressure over bony prominences.
  - Deliver a good seating posture on an appropriate pressure-relieving cushion in the wheelchair, with regular pressure relief and effective transfer technique.
- Heterotropic ossification (HO): The formation of normal lamellar bone in the soft tissues around paralysed joints below the level of the lesion; found to be present in around 4% to 20% of patients with SCI (Van Kuijik et al 2002). Surgical resection may be required.
- Syrinx and syringomyelia: A cavity filled with cerebrospinal fluid, which causes symptoms of pain, motor weakness and changes in spasticity. Most syrinx do not require surgical management, but it may be necessary to introduce a shunt to drain the fluid.

This chapter is an abridged version of Paddison and Hexter (2018) with permission.

References

ACPIN, 2014. Splinting for the prevention and correction of contractures in adults with neurological dysfunction. Available at: http://www.acpin.net/Downloads/Splinting_Guidelines/Splinting_Guidelines.pdf. (accessed 20.05.2018).

Alexander, M.S., Biering-Sorensen, F., Bodner, D., et al., 2009. International standards to document remaining autonomic function after spinal cord injury. Spinal Cord 47 (1), 36–43.

Amatachaya, S., Naewla, S., Srisim, K., Arrayawichanon, P., Siritaratiwat, W., 2014. Concurrent validity of the 10-meter walk test as compared with the 6-minute walk test in patients with spinal cord injury at various levels of ability. Spinal Cord 52 (4), 333–336.

Berg, K., 1993. Measuring Balance in the Elderly: Validation of an Instrument. (PhD thesis) McGill University, Canada.

Berlowitz, D.J., Tamplin, J., 2013. Respiratory muscle training for cervical spinal cord injury. Cochrane Database Systematic Review 23 (7), CD008507.

Bohannon, R.W., Smith, M.B., 1987. Interrater reliability of modified Ashworth scale of muscle spasticity. Physical Therapy 67 (2), 206–207.

Boninger, M.L., Brienza, D., Charllifus, S., Chen, Y.Y., et al., 2012. State of the science conference in spinal cord injury: introduction. Spinal Cord 50 (5), 342–343.

Borg, G.A., 1982. Psychophysical bases of perceived exertion. Medicine and Science in Sport and Exercise 14 (5), 377–381.

Brix Finnerup, N., 2013. Pain in patients with spinal cord injury. Pain 154, S71–S76.

Bromley, I., 2006. Tetraplegia and Paraplegia, sixth ed. Churchill Livingstone, London.

Bye, E.A., Harvey, L.A., Gambhir, A., et al., 2017. Strength training for partially paralysed muscles in people with recent spinal cord injury: a within-participant randomised controlled trial. Spinal Cord 55, 460–465.

Catz, A., Itzkovich, M., Tesio, L., et al., 2007. A multicenter international study on the spinal cord independence measure, version III: Rasch psychometric validation. Spinal Cord 45 (4), 275–291.

Curtis, K.A., Roach, K.E., Apllegate, E.B., et al., 1995. Development of the Wheelchair User's Shoulder Pain Index (WUSPI). Paraplegia 33 (2):290–293.

Curtis, K.A., Drysdale, G.A., Lanza, R.D., et al., 1999. Shoulder pain in wheelchair users with tetraplegia and paraplegia. Archives of Physical Medicine and Rehabilitation 80 (4):453–457.

Ditunno Jr., J.F., Cohen, M.E., Hauck, W.W., Jackson, A.B., Sipski, M.L., 2000. Recovery of upper extremity strength in complete and incomplete tetraplegia: a multicenter study. Archives of Physical Medicine and Rehabilitation 81 (4), 389–393.

Ditunno Jr., J.F., Scivoletto, G., Patrick, M., et al., 2008. Validation of the walking index for spinal cord injury in a US and European clinical population. Spinal Cord 46, 181–188.

Ditunno, P.L., Ditunno, J.F. Jr, 2001. Walking index for spinal cord injury (WISCI II): scale revision. Spinal Cord 39, 654–656.

Ditunno, J.F., Little, J.W., Tessler, A., Burns, A.S., 2004. Spinal shock revisited: a four-phase model. Spinal Cord 42, 383–395.

Field-Fote, E., Fluet, G., Schafer, S., et al., 2001. The spinal cord injury functional ambulation inventory (SCI-FAI). Journal of Rehabilitation Medicine 33, 177–181.

Foo, D., 1986. Spinal cord injury in forty four patients with cervical spondylosis. Paraplegia 24, 301–306.

Harvey, L.A., Glinsky, J.V., Bowden, J.L., 2016a. The effectiveness of 22 commonly administered physiotherapy interventions for people with spinal cord injury: a systematic review. Spinal Cord 54 (11), 914–923.

Harvey, L., 2016b. Physiotherapy rehabilitation for people with spinal cord injuries. Journal of Physiotherapy 62 (1), 4–11.

Harvey, L.A., Katalinic, O.M., Herbert, R.D., et al., 2017. Stretch for the treatment and prevention of contracture: an abridged republication of a Cochrane Systematic Review. Journal of Physiotherapy 63 (2), 67–75.

Holtz, K.A., Lipson, R., Noonan, V., et al., 2017. Prevalence and effect of problematic spasticity after traumatic spinal cord injury. Archives of Physical Medicine and Rehabilitation 98 (6), 1132–1138.

Chabra H.S. ISCoS Textbook on Comprehensive Management of Spinal Cord Injuries. Wolters Kluwer, New Delhi.

Johnston, L., 2001. Human spinal cord injury: new and emerging approaches to treatment. Spinal Cord 39, 609–613.

Karlsson, A.K., 2006. Autonomic dysfunction in spinal cord injury: clinical presentation of symptoms and signs. Progress in Brain Research 152:1–8.

Korse, N., Veldman, A., Peul, W., Vleggert-Lankamp, C., 2007. The long term outcome of micturition, defecation and sexual function after spinal surgery for cauda equina syndrome. PLoS One 12 (4):e0175987.

Linn, W.S., Spungen, A.M., Gong Jr., H., Adkins, R.H., Bauman, W.A., Waters, R.L., 2001. Forced vital capacity in two large outpatient populations with chronic spinal cord injury. Spinal Cord 39 (5), 263–268.

MacGregor, J., 1981. The evaluation of patient performance using long-term ambulatory monitoring technique in the domiciliary environment. Physiotherapy 67, 30–33.

Mateo, S., Roby-Brami, A., Reilly, K.T., et al., 2015. Upper limb kinematics after cervical spinal cord injury: a review. Journal of Neuroengineering and Rehabilitation 12, 9–12.

MASCIP Bowel Guidelines, 2012. Available at: www.mascip.co.uk/wp-content/uploads/2015/02/CV653N-Neurogenic-Guidelines-Sept-2012. (accessed 20.05.2018.).

MASCIP Standing Guidelinse, 2013. Available at: http://www.mascip.co.uk/wp-content/uploads/2015/05/Clinical-Guidelines-for-Standing-Adults-Following-Spinal-Cord-Injury.pdf.

MASCIP Turning Guidelines, 2015. Available at: https://www.mascip.co.uk/wp-content/uploads/2015/02/The-Patient-is-for-Turning-MASCIP-final-290813.pdf.

McKinley, W., Santos, K., Meade, M., Brooke, K., 2007. Incidence and outcomes of spinal cord injury clinical syndromes. Journal of Spinal Cord Medicine 30 (3), 215–224.

Nepomuceno, C., Fine, P.R., Richards, J.S., et al., 1979. Pain in patients with spinal cord injury. Archives of Physical Medicine and Rehabilitation 60, 605–609.

NHS England Service Standards, 2014. Standards for children and young people (<19 yrs) requiring spinal cord injury care. Available at: www.spinalcordinjury.nhs.uk/documents.

NICE, 2016. Spinal injury: assessment and initial management. Available at: www.nice.org.uk/guidance/ng41.

Paddison, S., Hexter, B., 2018. Spinal Cord Injury. In: Lennon, S., Ramdharry, G., Verheyden, G. (Eds.), Physical Management for Neurological Conditions, fourth ed. (Chapter 9) London.

Penn, R.D., Savoy, S.M., Corcos, D., et al., 1989. Intrathecal baclofen for severe spinal spasticity. The New England Journal of Medicine 320, 1517–1521, London.

Ptasinski, J., 2010. The effects of upper extremity Functional Electrically Stimulated (FES) exercise training on upper limb function in individuals with tetraplegia. ProQuest Dissertations and Theses. ProQuest Dissertations Publishing.

10

RISCI, 2017. Weaning Guidelines. Available at: http://risci.org.uk/weaning-guidelines-for-spinal-cord-injured-patients-in-critical-care-units.

SCI Action Canada, 2011. Physical activity guidelines for adults with a spinal cord injury. Available at: www.sciactioncanada.ca/docs/guidelines/Physical-Activity-Guidelines-for-Adults-with-a-Spinal-Cord-Injury-Health-Care-Professional.

Sheerin, F., 2005. Spinal cord injury: causation and pathophysiology. Emergency Nurse 12 (9), 29–38.

Schubert, V., Fagrell, B., 1991. Post occlusive reactive hyperemia and thermal response in the skin microcirculation of subjects with spinal cord injury. Scandinavian Journal of Rehabilitation Medicine 23 (1), 33–40.

Soleyman-Jahi, S., Yousefian, A., Maheronnaghsh, R., et al., 2017. Evidence-based prevention and treatment of osteoporosis after spinal cord injury: a systematic review. European Spinal Journal 1–17 May.

SCIFERTO Spinal Cord Injury Therapy Leads, 2016. Available at: mascip.co.uk.

Tator, C.H., 1998. Biology of neurological recovery and functional restoration after spinal cord injury. Neurosurgery 42 (2), 696–707.

Van Kuijik, A.A., Geurts, A.C., van Kuppevelt, H.J., 2002. Neurogenic heterotropic ossification in spinal cord injury. Spinal Cord 40 (7), 313–326.

Van Middendorp, J.J., Hosman, A.J., Donders, A.R., et al., 2011. A clinical prediction rule for ambulation outcomes after traumatic spinal cord injury: a longitudinal cohort study. Lancet 377 (9770), 1004–1010.

Van Straaten, M.G., Cloud, B.A., Zhao, K.D., Fortune, E., Morrow, M.M.B., 2017. Maintaining shoulder health after spinal cord injury: a guide to understanding treatments for shoulder pain. Archives of Physical Medicine and Rehabilitation 98 (5), 1061–1063.

Wyndaele, M., Wyndaele, J.J., 2006. Incidence, prevalence and epidemiology of spinal cord injury what learns a worldwide literature survey. Spinal Cord 44 (9), 523–529.

Whiteneck, G.G., Charlifue, S.W., Gerhart, K.A., Overhosler, J.D., Richardson, G.N., 1992. Quantifying handicap: a new measure of long-term rehabilitation outcomes. Archives of Physical Medicine and Rehabiliation 73, 519–526.

www.WHO.int, 2013. Available at: http://www.who.int/mediacentre/factsheets/fs384/en/

Useful websites

www.asia-spinalinjury.org/learning
www.elearnsci.org
www.iscos.org.uk
www.louisville.edu/medschool/neurosurgery/harkema/research/epiduralstimulation
www.nscisc.uab.edu
www.noigroup.com
www.nscisc.edu
www.physiotherapy exercises.com
www.rehabmeasure.com
www.scireproject.com

CHAPTER 11

Multiple sclerosis

Jennifer Freeman and Hilary Gunn

MULTIPLE SCLEROSIS

Multiple sclerosis (MS) is a chronic, progressive, demyelinating disease. It is the most common cause of nontraumatic neurological disability in young adults. The cause of MS is uncertain. It has a highly variable clinical presentation, which is dependent on lesion location and size.

TYPES OF MULTIPLE SCLEROSIS

The classification of disease subtype is highly relevant because of differences in prognosis (Freeman 2009) and because disease-modifying drugs are effective predominantly in people with relapse-remitting MS.

- Benign: One or two relapses with full recovery; in approximately 10% of cases (Coles 2009)
- Relapsing/remitting: With partial or complete recovery in between relapses; initial diagnosis of approximately 80% of cases, with approximately 65% of these individuals ultimately entering a secondary progressive phase (Compston & Coles 2008)
- Secondary progressive: Slowly progressive deterioration with or without relapses
- Primary progressive: Progressive deficit without remission; applicable to 10% to 15% of cases at onset

EPIDEMIOLOGY

- Affects approximately 2.5 million individuals worldwide (Compston & Coles 2008)
- Peaks between 20 and 40 years
- 3:1 ratio of females to males (Harbo 2013)
- Environmental factors appear to trigger an autoimmune reaction against central nervous system (CNS) myelin in genetically susceptible individuals (Kamm et al 2014)

DIAGNOSIS

- Multiple episodes of demyelination, which are separate in both time and lesion location within the CNS (McDonald et al 2001, Polman et al 2011).

PATHOLOGY
Demyelination

- Immune-mediated destruction of myelin producing characteristic lesions (plaques) throughout the CNS
- Widespread deficits throughout the white matter

Axonal Degeneration

- Scarring at the site of inflammatory plaques
- Axonal degeneration leading to residual disability

SYMPTOMS
Early

- Fatigue (lack of energy)
- Aching limbs
- Sensory disturbances
- Blurred or double vision

Sensory

- Numbness
- Paraesthesia
- Dysaesthesia

Motor

- Weakness
- Increased tone

Visual

- Acute optic neuritis with visual loss
- Diplopia (double vision)
- Nystagmus (rapid, repetitive eye movement in one direction, alternating with a slower movement in the opposite direction)

Vestibular

- Vertigo (false sensation of movement)

Cognitive

- Slowed information processing speed, impaired memory and executive function

Mood
● Depression

Cerebellar
● Unsteadiness
● Ataxia (disturbance in the coordination of movement)
● Nystagmus (defined later); intention tremor
● Slurred speech

Spinal Cord
● Spastic paresis with bowel and bladder disturbance and sexual dysfunction

PROGNOSIS
● Varies depending on MS subtype, age of onset and the areas of the CNS that are affected (Table 11.1) (Bergamaschi 2007).
● About 50% of patients are unable to walk without assistance 15 years after onset (Giesser 2011).

KEY NEEDS AT DIFFERENT STAGES OF MULTIPLE SCLEROSIS
The key needs and main focus of rehabilitation throughout the course of the disease change. It is helpful to divide the condition into four stages according to level of disability (Zajicek et al 2003).

Diagnosis Stage
● Appropriate support
● Access to information
● Continuing education
● Disease-modifying drugs

Table 11.1 Prognostic factors in multiple sclerosis

Factors associated with a relatively good outcome	Factors associated with a worse outcome
● Female	● Male
● Initial presentation of optic neuritis	● Initial presentation includes balance and walking problems
● Mainly sensory signs and symptoms	● Cerebellar and pyramidal symptoms
● Low relapse frequency	● High frequency of relapses
● Lack of problems in coordination and walking	● Progressive disease
● Low level of lesions on magnetic resonance imaging (MRI)	● High level of lesions on MRI

Adapted from Zajicek et al 2007.

Minimal Impairment Stage

● Advice, support and information
● Treatment of relapses
● Disease-modifying drugs
● Management of symptoms

Moderate Disability Stage

● Rehabilitation and symptomatic management
● Easy access to well-coordinated services
● Clear and consistent communication

Severe Disability Stage

● Good communication and coordinated care within the community
● Access to information and expertise
● Palliative and respite care (Oliver et al 2016)

MEDICAL MANAGEMENT

There is no definitive test for MS. People will often have undergone a range of investigations and a period of uncertainty before a diagnosis is confirmed.

Three main types of medical management:

● Disease-modifying therapies – treatments that aim to alter the disease course itself. These are predominantly effective in people with relapse-remitting MS.
● Short courses of oral or intravenous corticosteroids – treatments that aim to manage relapses. Evidence suggests steroids can help speed up recovery after a relapse.
● Treatments to help manage the symptoms associated with MS.

ASSESSMENT

The nature of MS means that a large range of clinical signs and symptoms may be experienced by each person. A collaborative and coordinated multi-disciplinary teamwork approach is essential. The unpredictable and fluctuating nature of MS means that assessment cannot be a one-off process. UK Clinical Guidelines (NICE 2014a) recommend at least an annual review to assess peoples needs (Table 11.2).

Table 11.2 Key assessment information for people with multiple sclerosis

Database
For newly diagnosed patients ● Confirmation of diagnosis: a second neurological event is required for confirmation of diagnosis ● Awareness of diagnosis: the neurologist or general practitioner should convey the diagnosis – not the physiotherapist

Table 11.2 Key assessment information for people with multiple sclerosis—cont'd

For people with established MS

● Classification of MS: benign, relapsing-remitting, primary progressive, secondary progressive (Pohlman 2011)

● Currently in relapse, or have they recently had a relapse? If so, how long ago was the relapse?

● Currently on a course of steroids? What is the steroid regimen?

● On disease-modifying drug therapy (e.g. beta interferons)?

● Using complementary medicine?

Subjective

Since you were last assessed, has any activity you used to undertake been limited, stopped or affected (NICE 2014a)?

Are there any other new problems that you think may be caused by MS that concern you? The therapist may need to give prompts regarding hidden symptoms (e.g. thinking, etc.)

● Mobility

● Balance and falling

● Control of your movements

● Bowel and bladder control

● Painful sensations

● Thinking

● Remembering

● Vision

● Mood (30%–50% of people with MS will develop major depression or anxiety at some point) (Marrie et al 2015)

Specific questions for people with a relapse

● How quickly are they recovering?

● How are they coping with these sudden changes?

● If the patient is currently on or has recently been on steroids, how have they responded to them?

Objective

Identify underlying impairments.

● Ataxia occurs in 80% of people with MS (Mills 2007).

● Fatigue (Rudroff 2016); two thirds of people report this as one of their most troubling symptoms (Induruwa 2012)

● Falls

● Balance
  Impaired balance is an important contributor to mobility difficulties and is associated with falls (Gunn et al 2014).

Continued

Table 11.2 Key assessment information for people with multiple sclerosis—cont'd

- Pain
  Experienced by an estimated 60% of people with MS (Foley 2013).
- Spasticity
  Experienced by up to 90% of people with MS (Rizzo et al 2004).
- Respiratory dysfunction
  Respiratory muscle weakness, bulbar dysfunction and associated cough impairments can result in respiratory problems (Gosselink et al 2000, Levy et al 2017).
  - Bladder and bowel control; up to 80% of people experience these problems at some time (Nortvedt et al 2007).

Identify activity limitations and participation restrictions.

- Mobility and gait
- Transfer ability and safety
- Daily functional activities
- Occupational issues; identify whether any physical problems (motor, sensory, fatigue) affect work ability
- Leisure pursuits
- Driving status

MS-Specific Tools

- The 12-item Multiple Sclerosis Walking Scale Version 2.0 (Hobart et al 2003)
- Multiple Sclerosis Impact Scale-29 Version 2.0 (Hobart et al 2001)
- Fatigue Scale for Motor and Cognitive Functions (Penner 2009)
- Multiple Sclerosis Quality of Life-54 Instrument (Vickrey et al 1995)
- Brief International Cognitive Assessment for Multiple Sclerosis (Langdon 2012)

Adapted from Freeman 2009 with permission.

REHABILITATION

UK Clinical Guidelines (NICE 2014a) advocate comprehensive, flexible and responsive review and reassessment systems to ensure ongoing support is available for people with MS and their carers. See management principles Box 11.1.

- Avoid crisis management.
- Focus on modifiable impairments (such as weakness, spasticity, deconditioning, pain and emotional distress) where these are identified as the primary contributors to functional limitations.
- Impaired balance is an important contributor to mobility difficulties and is often associated with falls (Gunn et al 2014).
- Consider cognitive impairments, which affect up to 50% of people with MS (Marrie et al 2015). The domains most frequently involved are information processing speed, memory and executive function (Feinstein et al 2015).
- Consider maintenance or slowing of deterioration as a positive outcome.
- Consider provision of adaptive equipment and modifications to the environment in a sensitive manner. These visible signs of growing disability are often rejected by patients.

- Consider reducing fatigue by energy conservation, exercise and cognitive behavioural approaches (Asano & Finlayson 2014).
- Consider respiratory problems: respiratory muscle weakness, bulbar dysfunction and associated cough impairments (Gosselink et al 2000, Levy et al 2017).
- Bladder and bowel symptoms are common in MS, with up to 80% of people experiencing problems at some time; refer to other professionals (Norvedt et al 2007).

Box 11.1 Key principles of management (from Freeman 2009 with permission)

Comprehensive assessment and ongoing review

Listening to and learning from patients

Ensuring the patient and the family are central to planning and participating in their own management

Clarifying the patient's perception of their main problems, their aims and expectations of interventions

Promoting self-management

Focusing therapy on maintaining activities within the context of the person's lifestyle

Offering ongoing support with flexible service provision and intensive rehabilitation as appropriate at different times

Adopting a coordinated multidisciplinary approach to management across services in various settings

PHYSIOTHERAPY INTERVENTIONS

The approach to management can be viewed in three ways as:

- health promotion (supporting people to incorporate exercise and physical activity into their lifestyle);
- restorative rehabilitation;
- maintenance rehabilitation.

The aim of physiotherapy is to:

- optimise physical activity;
- optimise functional ability and enhance participation (e.g. activities of daily living, work, social activities);
- target modifiable impairments (e.g. weakness, deconditioning, balance);
- optimise safe mobility; this includes appropriate assessment, provision and monitoring, as well as education about appropriate use of assistive devices and mobility aids, and involves the prevention and management of falls;
- Maintain comfortable and functional postures for sleeping, sitting and standing;

- support caregivers, whose needs are often overlooked (Borreani et al, 2014); this can be compounded by the fact that carers themselves may reject offers of support (Davies et al 2015);
- Prevent secondary complications, which can significantly affect function and quality of life.

Evidence for physiotherapy (interventions in alphabetical order):

Ataxia management

- Ataxia is very challenging to manage, and none of the available treatments are particularly effective (Marquer et al 2014, Marsden et al 2011).
  Consider recommendations for health care professionals on the management of people with ataxia published by Ataxia UK (2016).

Balance training

- Systematic reviews suggest that physiotherapy has generally small, but significant, beneficial effects on balance in people with mild to moderate disability (Campbell et al 2016, Paltamaa et al 2012).

Falls prevention and management

- An estimated 70% of people with MS fall each year (Nilsagard et al 2014). The causes of falls are multifactorial and the impacts are significant, including injury, activity curtailment and loss of independence. Research investigating interventions in this area is currently limited, but there is preliminary evidence of the effectiveness of education and support to optimise safe mobility and programmes of individualised, challenging, balance, gait and functional training (Carling et al 2016, Gunn et al 2015).

Fatigue management

- Rehabilitation interventions such as exercise, energy conservation treatment, vestibular rehabilitation and advice on healthy living (nutritional diet, regular sleeping patterns) have demonstrated some benefit, as has a cognitive behavioural educational approach (Asano & Finlayson 2014, Blikman et al 2013, Heine et al 2015).

Prevention of secondary complications

- Sixty per cent have contracture in at least one joint, with this being most common in the ankle joint; these are more common in people with progressive disease and in those who are more severely disabled (Hoang et al 2014). Stretching regimens, active exercise, splinting, functional electrical stimulation and standing programmes have demonstrated some benefit in maintaining joint range (Buchanan & Hourihan 2016).
- Approximately 15% of people with MS will develop a pressure ulcer at some point in the disease course (Cramp et al 2004). Assessment and monitoring are essential, particularly in people with more severe disability. Pressure-relieving equipment, postural management and effective moving and handling procedures are key to prevention and management.

Self-management and self-efficacy

● Ensure people have the skills, resources and strategies (such as identifying barriers and problem solving) to optimise successful long-term engagement in exercise and physical activity (Geidl et al 2014).

Spasticity management

● Identify and alleviate factors that may trigger or worsen spasticity. Refer to Buchanan and Hourihan (2016) for a comprehensive overview.

Strength training, aerobic conditioning and physical activity

● Physiotherapists should focus also on supporting people to be less sedentary and to undertake regular physical activity and exercise. There is strong evidence to support guidelines that recommend people with mild to moderate disability should aim to undertake 30 minutes of moderate-intensity aerobic exercise (e.g. stationary bicycle, treadmill or rowing machine) and 30 minutes of moderate-intensity strength training for major muscle groups twice a week (Latimer-Cheung et al 2013). Exercise is not detrimental to fatigue and may also have a positive impact on primary CNS damage by reducing inflammation and encouraging neuronal repair (Dalgas & Stenager 2012).

Upper limb training

● Target upper limb movement, and function with task-oriented training, constraint-induced therapy, strengthening and sensory reeducation training (Lamers et al 2016), as well as adjunct technologies (Taylor & Griffin 2015).

This chapter is an abridged version adapted from Freeman and Gunn (2018) with permission.

References

Asano, M., Finlayson, M.L., 2014. Meta-analysis of three different types of fatigue management interventions for people with multiple sclerosis: exercise, education, and medication. Multiple Sclerosis International 2014:798285.

Ataxia, U.K., 2016. Management of the Ataxias: Towards Best Clinical Practice, third ed. Ataxia UK, London.

Bergamaschi, R., 2007. Prognostic factors in multiple sclerosis. International Review of Neurobiology 79, 423–447.

Blikman, L.J., Huisstede, B.M., Kooijmans, H., Stam, H.J., Bussmann, J.B., van Meeteren, J., 2013. Effectiveness of energy conservation treatment in reducing fatigue in multiple sclerosis: a systematic review and meta-analysis. Archives of Physical Medicine and Rehabilitation 94, 1360–1376.

Borreani, C., Bianchi, E., Pietrolongo, E., Rossi, I., Cilia, S., et al., 2014. Unmet needs of people with severe multiple sclerosis and their carers: qualitative findings for a home-based intervention. PLoS ONE 9 (10), e109679.

Buchanan, K., Hourihan, S., 2016. Physical and postural management of spasticity (pages 57–82). In: Stevenson, V.L., Jarrett, L. (Eds.), Spasticity Management: A Practical Multidisciplinary Guide. CRC Press, London.

Campbell, E., Coulter, E.H., Mattison, P.G., Miller, L., McFadyen, A., Paul, L., 2016. Physiotherapy rehabilitation for people with progressive multiple sclerosis: a systematic review. Archives of Physical Medicine and Rehabilitation 97 (1), 141–151.

Carling, A., Forsberg, A., Gunnarsson, M., Nilsagard, Y., 2016. CoDuSe group exercise programme improves balance and reduces falls in people with multiple sclerosis: a multicentre, randomized, controlled pilot study. Multiple Sclerosis Journal 23 (10), 1394–1404.

Coles, A., 2009. Multiple sclerosis. Practical Neurology 9, 118–126.

Compston, A., Coles, A., 2008. Multiple sclerosis. Lancet 372, 1502–1517.

Cramp, A.F.L., Warke, K., Lowe-Strong, A.S., 2004. The incidence of pressure ulcers in people with multiple sclerosis and persons responsible for their management. International Journal of MS Care. 6 (2), 52–54.

Dalgas, U., Stenager, E., 2012. Exercise and disease progression in multiple sclerosis: can exercise slow down the progression of multiple sclerosis? Therapeutic Advances in Neurological Disorders 5 (2), 81–95.

Davies, F., Edwards, A., Brain, K., Edwards, M., Jones, R., Wallbank, R., et al., 2015. 'You are just left to get on with it': qualitative study of patient and carer experiences of the transition to secondary progressive multiple sclerosis. BMJ Open 5 (7), e007674.

Feinstein, A., Freeman, J., Lo, A.C., 2015. Treatment of progressive multiple sclerosis: what works, what does not, and what is needed. Lancet Neurology 14 (2), 194–207.

Foley, P.L., Vesterinen, H.M., Laird, B.J., et al., 2013. Prevalence and natural history of pain in adults with multiple sclerosis: systematic review and meta-analysis. Pain 154, 632–642.

Freeman, J.A., 2009. The patient with degenerative disease: multiple sclerosis. In: Lennon, S., Stokes, M. (Eds.), Pocketbook of Neurological Physiotherapy, first ed. Churchill Livingstone, Elsevier, Edinburgh.

Freeman, J.A., Gunn, H., 2018. Multiple Sclerosis. In: Lennon, S., Ramdharry, G., Verheyden, G. (Eds.), Physical Management for Neurological Conditions, fourth ed. Elsevier Science, London (Chapter 10).

Geidl, W., Semrau, J., Pfeifer, K., 2014. Health behaviour change theories: contributions to an ICF-based 8 behavioural exercise therapy for individuals with chronic diseases. Disability and Rehabilitation 36 (24), 2091–2100. 9.

Giesser, B.S.E., 2011. Primer on Multiple Sclerosis. Oxford University Press.

Gosselink, R., Kovacs, L., Ketelaer, P., Carton, H., Decramer, M., 2000. Respiratory muscle weakness and respiratory muscle training in severely disabled multiple sclerosis patients. Archives of Physical Medicine and Rehabilitation 81 (6), 747–751.

Gunn, H., Creanor, S., Haas, B., Marsden, J., Freeman, J., 2014. Frequency, characteristics and consequences of falls in multiple sclerosis: findings from a cohort study. Archives of Physical Medicine and Rehabilitation 95, 538–545.

Gunn, H., Markevics, S., Haas, B., Marsden, J., Freeman, J., 2015. Systematic review: the effectiveness of interventions to reduce falls and improve balance in adults with multiple sclerosis. Archives of Physical Medicine and Rehabilitation 96 (10), 1898–1912.

Harbo, H.F., Gold, R., Tintore, M., 2013. Sex and gender issues in multiple sclerosis. Therapeutic Advances in Neurological Disorders 6 (4), 237–248.

11

Heine, M., van de Port, I., Rietberg, M.B., van Wegen, E.E., Kwakkel, G., 2015. Exercise therapy for fatigue in multiple sclerosis. Cochrane Database of Systematic Reviews (9), CD009956.

Hoang, P.D., Gandevia, S.C., Herbert, R.D., 2014. Prevalence of joint contractures and muscle weakness in people with multiple sclerosis. Disability and Rehabilitation 36 (19), 1588–1593.

Hobart, J., Lamping, D., Fitzpatrick, R., Riazi, A., Thompson, A., 2001. The Multiple Sclerosis Impact Scale (MSIS-29): a new patient-based outcome measure. Brain 124, 962–973.

Hobart, J.C.J., Riazi, A., Lamping, D.L.D., Fitzpatrick, R., Thompson, A.J.A., 2003. Measuring the impact of MS on walking ability - The 12-Item MS Walking Scale (MSWS-12). Neurology 60, 31–36.

Induruwa, I., Constantinescu, C.S., Gran, B., 2012. Fatigue in multiple sclerosis - a brief review. Journal of the Neurological Sciences 323 (1–2), 9–15.

Kamm, C.P., Uitdehaag, B.M., Polman, C.H., 2014. Multiple sclerosis: current knowledge and future outlook. European Neurology 72, 132–141.

Langdon, D.W., Amato, M.P., Boringa, J., Brochet, B., Foley, F., Fredrikson, S., Hämäläinen, P., Hartung, H.P., Krupp, L., Penner, I.K., Reder, A.T., Benedict, R.H., 2012. Recommendations for a brief international cognitive assessment for multiple sclerosis (BICAMS). Multiple Sclerosis 18 (6), 891–898.

Lamers, I., Maris, A., Severijns, D., Dielkens, W., Geurts, S., Van Wijmeersch, B., et al., 2016. Upper limb rehabilitation in people with multiple sclerosis: a systematic review. Neurorehabilitation and Neural Repair 30 (8), 773–793.

Latimer-Cheung, A.E., Pilutti, L.A., Hicks, A.L., Martin Ginis, K.A., Fenuta, A.M., MacKibbon, K.A., et al., 2013. Effects of exercise training on fitness, mobility, fatigue, and health-related quality of life among adults with multiple sclerosis: a systematic review to inform guideline development. Archives of Physical Medicine and Rehabilitation 94 (9), 1800–1828. e3.

Levy, J., Bensmaila, D., Brotier-Chomiennea, A., Butelc, S., Joussaina, C., Hugerona, C., 2017. Respiratory impairment in multiple sclerosis: a study of respiratory function in wheelchair-bound patients. European Journal of Neurology 24 (3), 497–502 2017.

Marquer, A., Barbieri, G., Perennou, D., 2014. The assessment and treatment of postural disorders in cerebellar ataxia: a systematic review. Annals of Physical and Rehabilitation Medicine 57 (2), 67–78.

Marrie, R.A., Cohen, J., Stuve, O., Trojano, M., Sorensen, P.S., Reingold, S., et al., 2015. A systematic review of the incidence and prevalence of comorbidity in multiple sclerosis: overview. Multiple Sclerosis 21 (3), 263–281.

Marsden, J., Harris, C., 2011. Cerebellar ataxia: pathophysiology and rehabilitation. Clinical Rehabilitation 25, 195–216.

McDonald, W.I., Compston, A., Edan, G., Goodkin, D., Hartung, H.-P., Lublin, F.D., et al., 2001. Recommended diagnostic criteria for multiple sclerosis: guidelines from the international panel on the diagnosis of multiple sclerosis. Annals of Neurology 50, 121–127.

Mills, R.J., Yap, L., Young, C.A., 2007. Treatment for ataxia in multiple sclerosis. Cochrane Database of Systematic Reviews 1, CD005029.

National Institute for Clinical Excellence, 2014(a). Multiple sclerosis: management of multiple sclerosis in primary and secondary care. Clinical Guidelines-8, NICE. Available at: http://www.nice.org.uk.

Nilsagard, Y., Gunn, H., Freeman, J., Hoang, P., Lord, S., Mazumder, R., et al., 2014. Falls in people with MS: an individual data meta-analysis from studies from Australia, Sweden, United Kingdom and the United States. Multiple Sclerosis Journal 21 (1), 1–9.

Nortvedt, M.W., Riise, T., Frugaård, J., Mohn, J., Bakke, A., Skår, A.B., et al., 2007. Prevalence of bladder, bowel and sexual problems among multiple sclerosis patients two to five years after diagnosis. Multiple Sclerosis 13, 106–112.

Oliver, D.J., Borasio, G.D., Caraceni, A., de Visser, M., Grisold, W., Lorenzl, S., et al., 2016. A consensus review on the development of palliative care for patients with chronic and progressive neurological disease. European Journal of Neurology 23 (1), 30–38.

Paltamaa, J., Sjogren, T., Peurala, S.H., Heinonen, A., 2012. Effects of physiotherapy interventions on balance in multiple sclerosis: a systematic review and meta-analysis of randomized controlled trials. Journal of Rehabilitation Medicine 44 (10), 811–823.

Penner, I., Raselli, C., Stöcklin, M., Opwis, K., Kappos, L., Calabrese, P., 2009. The Fatigue Scale for Motor and Cognitive Functions (FSMC): validation of a new instrument to assess multiple sclerosis-related fatigue. Multiple Sclerosis Journal 15, 1509–1517.

Polman, C.H., Reingold, S.C., Banwell, B., Clanet, M., Cohen, J.A., Filippi, M., et al., 2011. Diagnostic criteria for multiple sclerosis: 2010 revisions to the McDonald criteria. Annals of Neurology 69, 292–302.

Rudroff, T., Kindred, J.H., Ketelhut, N.B., 2016. Fatigue in multiple sclerosis: misconceptions and future research directions. Frontiers in Neurology 7, 122. http://doi.org/10.3389/fneur.2016.00122.

Rizzo, M.A., Hadjimichael, O.C., Preiningerova, J., Vollmer, T.L., 2004. Prevalence and treatment of spasticity reported by multiple sclerosis patients. Multiple Sclerosis 10 (5), 589–595.

Taylor, M., Griffin, M., 2015. The use of gaming technology for rehabilitation in people with multiple sclerosis. Multiple Sclerosis Journal 21, 355–371.

Vickrey, B.G., Hays, R.D., Harooni, R., Myers, L.W., Ellison, G.W., 1995. A health-related quality of life measure for multiple sclerosis. Quality of Life Research 4, 187–206.

Zajicek, J., Freeman, J.A., Porter, B., 2007. Multiple Sclerosis Care: a Practical Manual. Oxford University Press, Oxford.

CHAPTER 12

Parkinson's

Bhanu Ramaswamy and Mariella Graziano

PARKINSON'S

Parkinson's is the second most common neurodegenerative disease worldwide. The cause is uncertain. People with Parkinson's present with a range of motor and nonmotor symptoms affecting automatic function, activity, participation and quality of life.

Types of Parkinson's

Parkinsonism is the umbrella term used to group people with similar characteristics (Goedert et al 2017):

- About 70% of people with parkinsonism have idiopathic Parkinson's, meaning the cause remains unknown.
- The remainder have atypical parkinsonism.

Epidemiology

- Global incidence ranges from 12 to 230 per 100,000 per year (Hirsch et al 2016).
- Parkinson's is more regularly diagnosed in the elderly, affecting around 1% of people over 65; however, increasingly, Parkinson's is being diagnosed in those under age 40 years (Bridgeman & Arsham 2017, p. 51).
- Parkinson's is more common in males, with a male/female ratio of 1.5:1 but with women typically living longer, numbers even out over time (Hirsch et al 2016).

Diagnosis

- The diagnosis of Parkinson's is typically based on motor symptoms and response to medication (Pagán 2012).
- Nonmotor symptoms like depression, constipation, psychosis, falls and sleep disturbances aid the diagnostic decision-making process (Chaudhuri et al 2006).

Pathology

- Motor symptoms in people with Parkinson's are predominantly associated with neurodegeneration in parts of the basal ganglia, a collection of nuclei in the subcortical region of the cerebrum and ventral midbrain, which is inter-related with surrounding central nervous system structures (Lanciego et al 2012).

● Depletion of the neurotransmitter dopamine in the substantia nigra of the basal ganglia causes compensatory changes in the basal ganglia pathways and leads to typical Parkinson's symptomatology affecting automatic movement quality (Pavese & Brooks 2009).

Symptoms

Key motor symptoms of Parkinson's are:

● Bradykinesia, characterised as slowness (at initiation of and during movement) and hypokinesia (reduced movement amplitude) of repeated movements, typically observed in writing, facial expression and arm swing during walking, but also present in any movement.

● Rigidity, being 'slowness to passive movements of major joints with the patient in a relaxed position and the examiner manipulating the limbs and neck (Goetz et al 2008). Resistance is velocity independent and often tested through flexion and extension movements.

● Resting tremor of 4 to 6 Hz, usually becoming inhibited when initiating movement. Frequently present as a reciprocal movement of thumb and forefinger, called *pill-rolling tremor.*

● Not seen at diagnosis, but later in the course is postural instability, creating high falls risk, in part from the 'stooped posture' that results from weakness in antigravity muscles and changes in muscle tone leading to lack of adequate postural adjustments and thus balance deficits.

Gait alterations in people with Parkinson's comprise:

● shuffling gait, typically with short, close steps and reduced foot clearance;

● festination by centre of mass falling relatively forward to the base of support and leading to increased step frequency but reduced amplitude;

● freezing, which is seen as further descaled, hesitant steps, with poor ability to prepare and sustain movement, especially when attention is compromised.

Nonmotor symptoms include:

● sleep disorders such as from restless legs, rapid eye movement (REM) sleep disturbance, insomnia or daytime sleepiness;

● autonomic disturbances like bladder and sexual dysfunction, excessive sweating or orthostatic hypotension;

● gastrointestinal dysfunction, including dribbling, swallowing problems, nausea or constipation;

● sensory symptoms comprising pain, paraesthesia or olfactory impairment;

- neuropsychiatric features such as depression, anxiety, apathy, cognitive disorders, hallucinations or delusions;
- others such as fatigue, visual disturbance and weight loss or gain.

Prognosis
- There is some evidence that people with Parkinson's have reduced life expectancy (Ishihara et al 2007).
- The increased risk of a respiratory complication is linked with mortality in people with Parkinson's (Pennington et al 2010).
- Higher mortality risk is also significantly associated with age at onset, severity of motor symptoms, cognitive impairment and dementia, and psychotic symptoms (Aarsland et al 2008; Forsaa et al 2010).

Medical Management
The focus of medical management of people with Parkinson's is on pharmacological interventions:
- Dopaminergic medications that increase the dopamine availability in the brain are the standard drug therapies (Hornykiewicz 2017).
- Nondopaminergic (e.g. tremor-reducing drugs) are used as well, as is medication for nonmotor symptoms.
- People with Parkinson's with sustained use of antiparkinsonian medication are typically seen with abnormal involuntary movement and fluctuating on (medication-improved motor symptoms) and off (ineffective symptomatic control) periods or psychiatric disorders such as hallucinations or psychosis.

For a selected group of people with Parkinson's, deep brain stimulation is recommended, whereby a surgical procedure implants a continuous stimulator to alleviate motor symptoms. Nevertheless, people with Parkinson's continue to show a decline in activities of daily living consistent with the progression of the disease process.

Assessment
See Table 12.1.

Rehabilitation
- The overall goal should be to enable people to be active, engaged and participating in (social) activities, thereby enhancing quality of life (Keus et al 2014).
- Management is about symptomatic control, which is best delivered by professionals with expertise in Parkinson's working together via multidisciplinary teams (Bloem & Munneke 2014).

- Being diagnosed with a degenerative disorder requires honest but positive language (National Institute of Health and Care Excellence (NICE) 2017) towards the person with the condition and their surroundings. Communicate with people with Parkinson's through positive language with, 'shared-management' messages.
- A frequently used categorisation of people with Parkinson's seen in research, or used by medical colleagues includes the motor-defined stages such the Hoehn and Yahr scale (Hoehn & Yahr 1967), ranging from 1 to 5, with 1 representing unilateral involvement and 5 being confined to bed or chair.

Table 12.1 Key assessment information for people with Parkinson's

Database
Obtain medical information:
● Parkinson's diagnosis, year of diagnosis, medically described disease stage
● Motor complications
● Cognitive complications
● Pain
● Comorbidity
● Current (non)medical treatment
● Earlier treatment approaches, especially physiotherapy interventions of use
Collect external factors:
● Personal: age and gender; insight into the condition; coping
● Environmental: medication; assistive devices; family, living and carer information

Subjective
Ask for perceived problem:
● What is the most important problem (prioritise physiotherapy-relevant problems)?
● How is the carer involved in this?
What are the expectations of the person with Parkinson's?
● With regard to prognosis
● With regard to physiotherapy treatment
● With regard to shared management
Provide description of level of functioning and activities:
● Transfers
● Balance and (near) falls
● Manual dexterity
● Gait
● Physical capacity (include if mood is affecting participation in regular exercise)
Document participation: status of relationships, work and social life
Are there tips and tricks the person with Parkinson's uses as compensation for a problem, and are these strategies helpful?

12

Table 12.1 Key assessment information for people with Parkinson's—cont'd

Objective

Observe the person with Parkinson's when rising from the waiting room chair, walking into the treatment room, closing the door and taking off a coat.

Assess the following domains:

- Physical capacity and pain
  - Muscle strength and power
  - Muscle tone
  - Joint flexibility
  - Exercise performance and tolerance
  - Pain
- Transfers
  - Sit to stand, bed mobility, getting up from the floor, getting in and out of the car
  - Safety: fall or near fall
- Manual dexterity including reaching, grasping and moving objects
- Balance
  - During transfers, walking and dual tasking
  - Safety: fall or near fall
- Gait
  - Gait pattern impairments
  - Festination or freezing
  - Safety: fall or near fall
- Other
  - Respiratory strength, especially later in the condition

Parkinson's–specific tools

Measurement tools validated with a Parkinson's population for these domains are:

- Physical capacity
  - Six-minute walk test and Borg scale
  - Five times sit-to-stand
- Transfers
  - Modified Parkinson's activity scale: bed
  - Modified Parkinson's activity scale: chair
  - Timed up and go test
  - Five times sit-to-stand
- Manual dexterity
  - Nine-hole peg test
  - Purdue pegboard test
  - Manual ability measure (MAM-16)
- Balance
  - Push and release test
  - Mini-BESTest
  - Berg balance scale
- Gait
  - Modified Parkinson's activity scale: gait
  - Ten-metre walk test
  - Six-minute walk test
  - Dynamic gait index

Based on Keus et al 2014.

Physiotherapy Interventions (Tables 12.2 and 12.3, and for more detail see Ramaswamy & Graziano 2018)

Key physiotherapy strategies (based on current research evidence, but not exhaustive of clinical practice examples) presented according to Hoehn and Yahr stages are (Keus et al 2014):

- Stage 1:
  - Support shared management to monitor the condition themselves, but seek help as appropriate
  - Prevent inactivity through education and exercise
  - Prevent fear to move or fall

Table 12.2 Key interventions for people with Parkinson's

Modality	Description
Exercise (related to conditioning)	● To remain physically active, reduce discomfort when mobility is affected and continue to live a desired lifestyle. ● Introduce exercises to be carried out daily (NICE 2017). ● Exercise has also been shown to be beneficial in managing nonmotor symptoms (Speelman et al 2011) and reduces the risk of secondary complications, pain and fear of moving and falling. ● People with Parkinson's should develop an exercise-focused lifestyle beginning at the point of diagnosis (Parkinson's UK 2017). ● Body conditioning maximises fitness components in addition to targeting improvement in gait, balance, transfer and physical capacity. ● To be included are motor-cognitive (e.g. dual tasks) exercises as well as exergaming through the use of technology. ● Coach people with Parkinson's in finding ways to focus on disease-specific issues and allowing them to keep up the conditioning, including supporting others to assist the person with Parkinson's with exercise.

Practice (related to motor learning and performance)	● People with Parkinson's can still learn in a later phase, even if affected by their cognitive ability.
	● Motor learning principles such as task specificity, intensity, progression and feedback should be applied.
	● Practice aims to achieve a level of automaticity, which can be assessed by:
	  ● The response when carrying out a dual task and evaluating how much one task interferes with the other (automatisation)
	  ● Observing the ability to perform an untrained task with a similar context (transfer)
	  ● If the individual is able to retrieve performance after some time has passed (retention)

Movement strategies training	● People with Parkinson's can be taught to compensate where automatic movement is affected by cognitive impairment. ● Strategies include cueing and attention and strategies for complex motor sequences. ● Keep commands short and simple.

Table 12.3 Key evidence-based interventions for people with Parkinson's Enlisted are interventions with a positive, significant effect and subsequently either low to moderate quality of evidence (small effect or very large confidence interval) or moderate to high quality of evidence

Core area	Interventions
Balance	• Conventional physiotherapy improves basic balance and functional reach (low/moderate quality of evidence). • Treadmill training improves basic balance (low/moderate quality of evidence). • Cueing improves dynamic gait ability (low/moderate quality of evidence). • Dance (tango) improves basic and advanced balance (low/moderate quality of evidence). • Tai chi reduces number of falls, improves basic balance and functional reach (low/moderate quality of evidence).
Gait	• Conventional physiotherapy improves gait speed (moderate/high quality of evidence). • Treadmill training improves gait speed and stride length (moderate/high quality of evidence) and walking distance (low/moderate quality of evidence). • Cueing improves gait speed (moderate/high quality of evidence) and step length and reduces freezing of gait (low/moderate quality of evidence). • Strategies for complex movement sequences improve stride length (low/moderate quality of evidence). • Tai chi improves gait speed, stride length and walking distance (low/moderate quality of evidence).
Gait, balance and transfers	• Conventional physiotherapy improves timed up and go mobility (low/moderate quality of evidence). • Strategies for complex movement sequences improve Parkinson's activity level (moderate/high quality of evidence). • Dance (tango) improves timed up and go mobility (low/moderate quality of evidence). • Tai chi improves timed up and go mobility (low/moderate quality of evidence).
Transfers	• Cueing improves sit-to-stand ability (low/moderate quality of evidence). • Strategies for complex movement sequences improve chair transfers (moderate/high quality of evidence).
Physical capacity	• Conventional physiotherapy improves muscle strength (moderate/high quality of evidence). • Treadmill training improves walking distance (low/moderate quality of evidence). • Tai chi improves muscle strength and walking distance (low/moderate quality of evidence).
Other	• Conventional physiotherapy improves quality of life (low/moderate quality of evidence). • Massage improves patient-based treatment effect (low/moderate quality of evidence). • Strategies for complex movement sequences improve patient-based treatment effect (low/moderate quality of evidence).

Based on Keus et al 2014.

- ● Improve physical capacity
- ● Reduce pain
- ● Delay onset of activity limitations (up to stage 3)
- ● Stages 2 to 4:
  - ● In addition to the earlier mentioned interventions, maintain or reduce limitations in transfers, balance, manual activities and gait through practice and strategy training
- ● Stage 5:
  - ● In addition to the previously mentioned approaches, maintain vital functions (especially respiratory system), prevent pressure sores and contractures and support and coach carers and nurses

This chapter is an abridged version adapted from Ramaswamy and Graziano (2018) with permission.

References

Aarsland, D., Beye, M.E., Kreuz, M.W., 2008. Dementia in Parkinson's disease. Current Opinion in Neurology 21, 676–682.

Bloem, B., Munneke, M., 2014. Revolutionising management of chronic disease: the ParkinsonNet approach. BMJ 348, g1838. https://doi.org/10.1136/bmj.g1838.

Bridgeman, K., Arsham, T., 2017. The Comprehensive Guide to Parkinson's Disease. Viartis, London.

Chaudhuri, R., Healy, D., Schapira, A., 2006. Non-motor symptoms of Parkinson's disease: diagnosis and management. Lancet Neurology 5, 235–245.

Forsaa, E.B., Larsen, J.P., Wentzel-Larsen, T., et al., 2010. What predicts mortality in Parkinson disease? A prospective population-based long-term study. Neurology 75 (14), 1270–1276.

Goedert, M., Jakes, R., Spillantini, M.G., 2017. The synucleinopathies: twenty years on. Journal of Parkinson's Disease 7, S51–S69.

Goetz, C.G., Tilley, B.C., Shaftman S.R., et al., 2008. Movement disorder society-sponsored revision of the unified Parkinson's disease rating scale (mds-updrs): scale presentation and clinimetric testing results. Movement Disorders 23, 2129–2170.

Hirsch, L., Jette, N., Frolkis, A., et al., 2016. The incidence of Parkinson's disease: a systematic review and meta-analysis. Neuroepidemiology 46 (4), 292–300.

Hoehn, M.M., Yahr, M.D., 1967. Parkinsonism: onset, progression and mortality. Neurology 17 (5), 427–442.

Hornykiewicz, O., 2017. L-DOPA. Journal of Parkinson's Disease 7, S3–S10.

Ishihara, L., Cheesbrough, A., Brayne, C., et al., 2007. Estimated life expectancy of Parkinson's patients compared with the UK population. Journal of Neurology Neurosurgery Psychiatry 78, 1304–1309.

Keus, S.H.J., Munneke, M., Graziano, M., et al., 2014. European Physiotherapy Guideline for Parkinson's Disease. KNGF/ParkinsonNet, The Netherlands.

Lanciego, J., Luquin, N., Obeso, J., 2012. Functional neuroanatomy of the basal ganglia. Cold Spring Harb Perspect Medicine 2, a009621.

National Institute of Health and Care Excellence, 2017. Parkinson's Disease in Adults. NG71. NICE, London.

Pagán, F., 2012. Improving outcomes through early diagnosis of Parkinson's disease. American Journal of Managed Care 18, S176–S182.

Parkinson's UK, 2017. Exercise Framework for Parkinson's – in press.

Pavese, N., Brooks, D., 2009. Imaging neurodegeneration in Parkinson's disease. Biochimica et Biophysica Acta 1792, 722–729.

Pennington, S., Snell, K., Lee, M., et al., 2010. The cause of death in idiopathic Parkinson's disease. Parkinsonism and Related Disorders 16 (7), 434–437.

Ramaswamy, B., Graziano, M., 2018. Parkinson's. In: Lennon, S., Ramdharry, G., Verheyden, G. (Eds.), Physical Management for Neurological Conditions, fourth ed. Elsevier, London.

Speelman, A., Van de Warrenburg, B., Van Nimwegen, M., et al., 2011. How might physical activity benefit patients with Parkinson disease? Nature Reviews Neurology 7, 528–534.

CHAPTER 13

Guillain–Barré syndrome

Gita Ramdharry and Aisling Carr

GUILLAIN–BARRÉ SYNDROME

Guillain–Barré syndrome (GBS) is an umbrella term for acute-onset, inflammatory neuropathies. It is an acquired polyneuropathy caused by an acute episode of inflammation of the peripheral nerves, often after an infection. GBS is an autoimmune disorder where specific parts of the nerve are targeted by the body's own defence mechanisms. The classic presentation of GBS is a rapid onset of ascending limb paralysis and sensory impairment (van den Berg et al 2014, van Doorn 1983, Willison et al 2016).

TYPES OF GUILLAIN–BARRÉ SYNDROME

There are different forms and variants of GBS classified according to the type of nerve and part of the nerve affected:

● Acute inflammatory demyelinating polyradiculoneuropathy (AIDP) occurs where there is a patchy, inflammatory attack on the myelin along the length of the nerve at both proximal and distal ends. Both motor and sensory peripheral nerves are affected.

● Acute motor axonal neuropathy (AMAN) is a form where the motor axons are predominantly affected.

● Acute motor sensory axonal neuropathy (AMSAN) involves the axons of both motor and sensory nerves

● Miller–Fisher syndrome (MFS) is a variant of GBS where the cranial nerves are involved with a 'triad' presentation of ataxia, areflexia and ophthalmoplegia. MFS can overlap with GBS with a presentation of limb paralysis (Wakerley et al 2017).

EPIDEMIOLOGY

GBS is a rare, sporadically occurring disease, and incidence rates range from 0.35 to 1.34 per 100,000 each year (Lehmann et al 2012). It can affect any age group but is more prevalent in men and in older people, where the long-term outcome can be much worse (Vucic et al 2009). The most common form in Europe and North America is AIDP. In Asia, the AMAN and AMSAN forms are seen more frequently.

DIAGNOSIS

- History of acute, symmetrical and rapidly progressive limb weakness (Willison et al 2016, van den Berg et al 2014)
- Possible history or preceding infection and/or fever (Willison et al 2016, van den Berg et al 2014)
- Areflexia (Willison et al 2016, van den Berg et al 2014)
- Sensory impairment in limbs (in AIDP or AMSAN) (Willison et al 2016, van den Berg et al 2014)
- Abnormal nerve conduction studies:
  - AIDP: slowed nerve conduction velocity, indicating demyelination
  - AMAN or AMSAN: normal conduction velocity, but reduced size of the compound muscle action potential, indicating axonal loss (Vucic et al 2009)
- Elevated cerebrospinal fluid protein in 80% of cases with albuminocytological dissociation (fewer than 10 white cells) (Hughes 2008)
- Ganglioside antibodies in 25% of cases (Hughes 2008)

PATHOLOGY

GBS is an autoimmune disorder where an immune response is directed towards unknown antigens triggered by the earlier infection. In about two thirds of cases, the preceding infectious agent can be identified (Lehmann et al 2012, Vucic et al 2009); *Campylobacter Jejuni*, Cytomegalovirus, Epstein–Barr and influenza A viruses have been implicated (Willison et al 2016). In AIDP, the immune response to the original infection leads to an inflammatory process mediated by antibodies that cross-react with specific bacterial epitopes and similar proteins on the surface of neuronal myelin. This molecular mimicry leads to destruction of the myelin sheath and disruption of saltatory conduction leading to a slowing or block of nerve conduction (Fig. 13.1).

SYMPTOMS

The common signs and symptoms of GBS are outlined, but there will be some diversity among the different variants (Ali et al 2006, England & Asbury 2004, Lehmann et al 2012, Vucic et al 2009):

- Lower motor neurone weakness and hypotonia: ascending in the acute phase
- Sensory impairment: ascending numbness and paraesthesia in the acute phase
  - Large fibre sensory loss: pinprick, vibration and proprioception
- Areflexia
- Low back pain caused by nerve root inflammation
- Cranial nerve involvement in 50% of AIDP cases and MFS
  - Diplopia, facial and bulbar weakness
- Autonomic involvement: cardiac arrhythmias, fluctuations in blood pressure
- Fatigue

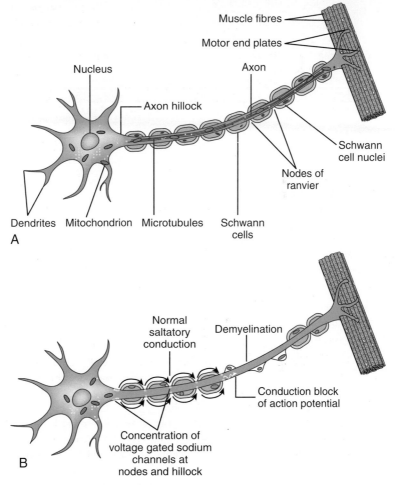

Fig. 13.1
(A) Normal motor neurone. (B) Acute demyelination and conduction block.

In severe cases of GBS, the following signs and symptoms may be observed:

● Trunk weakness
● Bulbar dysfunction
● Neuromuscular respiratory failure
● Vital capacity below 20 mL/kg
● Impaired cough

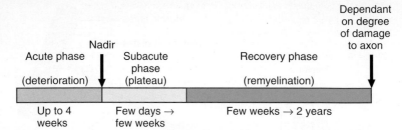

Fig. 13.2
Disease course for GBS.

DISEASE COURSE AND PROGNOSIS

GBS typically runs a monophasic course. Severity is variable, but in AIDP weakness reaches nadir within 4 weeks during the demyelination phase (Fig. 13.2) with recovery following as remyelination occurs. About 5% of patients initially diagnosed with GBS turn out to have chronic inflammatory demyelinating polyradiculoneuropathy (CIDP). Ten per cent to 20% of cases are left with disabling symptoms (Vucic et al 2009).

Factors associated with poor recovery:
● Higher degree of axonal damage during the early stages of the disease
● Higher degree of secondary axonal loss
● High levels of impairment at nadir
● Older age

MEDICAL MANAGEMENT

If mobility is not affected, management is conservative and recovery is gradual. In more severe cases, intravenous immunoglobulins (IVIg) and plasma exchange speed up recovery, but do not change the endpoint. They have been proven to have equal efficacy in the treatment of GBS when mobility is impaired (England & Asbury 2004).

Despite treatment, GBS can be a severe disease, as about 25% of patients require artificial ventilation during a period of days to months, about 20% of patients are still unable to walk after 6 months and 3% to 10% of patients die. In severely affected individuals, high-quality supportive care is paramount; ventilator and circulatory support is essential for those with significant respiratory failure or dysautonomia and must be managed in a critical care setting. Supported nutrition and protection against aspiration is part of managing those with bulbar involvement.

Table 13.1 Outcome measures for use in people with GBS and other immune-mediated neuropathies

Assessment	Measurement tool
Muscle strength	● MRC scale or Rasch modified MRC scale for immune-mediated neuropathy (Vanhoutte et al 2012) ● Handheld myometry (Schwid et al 1999)
Fatigue	● Fatigue Severity Scale for immune-mediated neuropathy (van Nes et al 2009)
Joint range of motion	● Goniometry
Pain	● Visual analogue scale
Composite physical functioning assessment	● Rasch-built Overall Disability Scale for immune-mediated neuropathy (van Nes et al 2011) ● Overall neuropathy limitation scale (Graham et al 2006a)
Walking	● Ten-metre timed walk (speed) and 6-minute walk (endurance) (Padua et al 2016) ● Walk-12 scale (perception of walking ability) (Graham et al 2006b)
Balance	● Berg Balance Scale and Tinetti Balance test (Monti Bragadin et al 2015) ● Modified Clinical Test of Sensory Integration and Balance (Shumway-Cook & Horak 1986)
Hand function	● Nine-hole peg test ● Functional dexterity test (Piscoquito et al 2012, Videler et al 2008)

MRC, Medical research council.

13

Medical management of pain includes simple analgesics; opioids but more often antidepressants such as gabapentin or amitriptyline are required to manage the neuropathic discomfort.

ASSESSMENT

Outlined are principles of assessment. Specific assessment tools and outcome measures are outlined in Table 13.1.

In the acute setting:
● Respiratory status: vital capacity, ventilatory requirements (if in critical care), presence of secondary respiratory complications (see Chapter 6)
● Daily assessment of joint range of motion to identify risks of soft tissue shortening
● Full assessment of muscle strength, if the person is awake, noting distribution and severity of weakness

- Sensory impairment: pinprick, light touch, joint position sense and vibration (tuning fork), noting the modality and distribution of impairment
- Skin integrity
- Pain and pain management
- Autonomic symptoms when moved or moving
- Social history
  In the rehabilitation phase:
- Expanded social history, emotional well-being and the person's expectations/aspirations of rehabilitation
- Muscle strength and sensory impairment to monitor improvement
- Functional ability: sitting, standing, balance, walking, upper limb function
- Fatigue severity and impact on function
- Pain

REHABILITATION AND PHYSIOTHERAPY APPROACHES

There is a small evidence base for rehabilitation approaches for people with GBS. Lessons can be learned, however, from other polyneuropathies with more established treatment approaches, for example, diabetic neuropathy or inherited neuropathies (Ramdharry et al 2018).

Rehabilitation in the Acute Phase

There are no studies on the efficacy of early rehabilitation approaches in GBS. At present intervention is based on experience with other neurological conditions, though the need for therapy input is recognised (Vucic et al 2009). Physical management in the acute stage focuses on respiratory interventions and prevention of secondary complications (Khan 2004) (Table 13.2). Respiratory treatments include sputum clearance techniques, maintenance of lung volumes and breathing exercises when the person is able to participate (see Chapter 6). Other interventions advocated are early mobilisation, splinting, positioning, stretches to maintain joint range of motion and exercises to increase strength and endurance (Hughes 2008, Khan 2012, Meythaler 1997). Fear, anxiety and sleep deprivation are common problems experienced by people with GBS in the early stages. Good two-way communication between the multidisciplinary team (MDT) and the patient and carers is vital to ensure they are informed at every stage. This may be challenging if a person is intubated, but it can be supported by speech and language therapy intervention.

Rehabilitation in the Subacute and Later Stages

Approximately 40% of all people with GBS will need a period of multidisciplinary inpatient rehabilitation with the aim of maximising functional recovery and participation (Khan 2012) (Table 13.2). A survey of 800 people with GBS found that

Table 13.2 Summary of treatment approaches for people in different phases of recovery from GBS

	Treatment approaches	Considerations
Acute stage of GBS	Respiratory interventions Positioning Splinting and stretching Early mobilisation Strength training	Rehabilitation approach and goals Communication if intubated Pain Fatigue
Rehabilitation stage and long-term management of GBS	Exercise: ● Aerobic exercise ● Strength training ● Stretching Balance training: ● Self-generated movements ● Reacting to perturbations ● Multisensory proprioceptive training ● Divided attention Orthotic management: ● Foot orthoses and insoles ● Off-the-shelf or custom-made ankle foot orthoses ● Vibrating insoles (when commercially available) Pain and fatigue management: ● Exercise ● Education ● Pacing ● MDT involvement (Occupational Therapy and psychology)	Subacute and early recovery phase: ● Rehabilitation approach and goals Later recovery and long term: ● Management approach and goals Delivery within self-management frameworks: ● Coaching to problem solve and make choices ● Facilitating exploration and taking action

GBS, Guillain–Barré syndrome; *MDT*, multidisciplinary team.

people who did not receive physiotherapy treatment as an outpatient or in the community had greater levels of disability than those who did (Davidson et al 2009).

Exercise and balance training. In a systematic review of exercise in people with inflammatory neuropathy (including CIDP), seven studies were identified that met the review criteria (Simatos et al 2016). Four were single case studies, and one was of exercise bike training that only assessed cardiopulmonary outcomes of the programme. Of the remaining two studies, one was of exercise bike training (Garssen et al 2004) and the other was a multidisciplinary, individualised rehabilitation intervention that included physiotherapy (strength, endurance and gait training), occupational therapy (work, community tasks) and counselling with a psychologist (Khan et al 2011). Twelve weeks of exercise bike training resulted in improved knee extensor strength and cardiopulmonary variables in 20 people with CIDP and GBS, but no additional measures of functional balance or mobility were included in this study (Garssen et al 2004). The multidisciplinary rehabilitation study included 79 participants in a randomised controlled trial (Khan et al 2011). Participants receiving the high-intensity rehabilitation intervention, which included strength, endurance and gait training, demonstrated significant improvements in the Functional Independence Measure (FIM). There were also significant improvements, with moderate effect sizes, in the mobility and locomotion domains of the FIM.

There is little evidence of the effectiveness of balance training in GBS, but lessons can be learned from a good evidence base in people with diabetic neuropathy. A systematic review of exercise interventions showed positive effects on static balance, gait and lower limb strength. The 10 trials included tested interventions such as tai chi, proprioceptive balance training, gait training and lower limb resistance training (Chapman et al 2017).

Orthotic interventions. Evidence for the effect of orthotics interventions is again extrapolated from trials in other polyneuropathies (Sackley et al 2009). The main purpose of orthotic intervention for people with GBS is to improve gait and balance through one or more of the following biomechanical aims:

● Redistribution of pressure under the foot
● Realignment and correction of foot deformities
● Reduction of foot drop
● Stabilisation of the ankle joint
● Increasing sensory feedback to the foot and/or ankle

In view of the limited evidence for the efficacy of orthotic provision, clinicians should review any devices prescribed with appropriate outcome measures, depending on the aim of the device. People with polyneuropathy may be reluctant to accept orthoses (O'Connor et al 2016, Phillips et al 2011, Ramdharry et al 2012a), so consideration of the person's opinion and inclusion in decision making will help ensure that a device is prescribed that is acceptable to that individual. Measures of comfort should also be recorded over time, as ill-fitting splints can be another reason for nonuse.

PAIN AND FATIGUE MANAGEMENT

Pain is a recognised issue that can adversely affect quality of life. Musculoskeletal pain may be ameliorated with physiotherapy interventions and neuropathic pain with drugs, but some people with GBS live with persistent pain. Pain management principles of education, exercise and support are beneficial. Referrals to multidisciplinary pain management programmes may be warranted, but have not been investigated as a specific approach in the polyneuropathy literature. Similarly, referrals to fatigue management by occupational therapy colleagues may be helpful. There are no specific interventional studies in any polyneuropathies, but anecdotally, people with other types of polyneuropathy report benefits in learning how to pace, use rest breaks and consider adaptive equipment to conserve energy (Ramdharry et al 2012b).

This chapter is an abridged version adapted from Ramdharry, Carr and Laurá (2018) with permission.

References

Ali, M.I., Fernández-Pérez, E.R., Pendem, S., Brown, D.R., Wijdicks, E.F.M., Gajic, O., 2006. Mechanical ventilation in patients with Guillain-Barré syndrome. Respiratory Care 51 (12), 1403–1407.

Chapman, A., Meyer, C., Renehan, E., Hill, K.D., Browning, C.J., 2017. Exercise interventions for the improvement of falls-related outcomes among older adults with diabetes mellitus: a systematic review and meta-analyses. Journal Diabetes Complications 31 (3), 631–645.

Davidson, I., Wilson, C., Walton, T., Brissenden, S., 2009. Physiotherapy and Guillain-Barré syndrome: results of a national survey. Physiotherapy 95 (3), 157–163.

England, J.D., Asbury, A.K., 2004. Peripheral neuropathy. Lancet 363 (9427), 2151–2161.

Garssen, M.P.J., Bussmann, J.B.J., Schmitz, P.I.M., Zandbergen, A., Welter, T.G., Merkies, I.S.J., et al., 2004. Physical training and fatigue, fitness, and quality of life in Guillain–Barré syndrome and CIDP. Neurology 63 (12), 2393–2395.

Graham, R.C., Hughes, R.A.C., 2006a. A modified peripheral neuropathy scale: the Overall Neuropathy Limitations Scale. Journal Neurology Neurosurg Psychiatry 77 (8), 973–976.

Graham, R.C., Hughes, R.A.C., 2006b. Clinimetric properties of a walking scale in peripheral neuropathy. Journal Neurology Neurosurg Psychiatry 77 (8), 977–979.

Hughes, R., 2008. Peripheral nerve diseases: the bare essentials. Practice. Neurology 8 (6), 396–405.

Khan, F., 2004. Rehabilitation in Guillian Barre syndrome. Australian Family Physician 33 (12), 1013–1017.

Khan, F., Amatya, B., 2012. Rehabilitation interventions in patients with acute demyelinating inflammatory polyneuropathy: a systematic review. European Journal Physiology Rehabiliation Medicine 48 (3), 507–522.

Khan, F., Pallant, J., Amatya, B., Ng, L., Gorelik, A., Brand, C., 2011. Outcomes of high- and low-intensity rehabilitation programme for persons in chronic phase after Guillain-Barré syndrome: a randomized controlled trial. Journal Rehabilition Medicine 43 (7), 638–646.

Lehmann, H.C., Hughes, R.A.C., Kieseier, B.C., Hartung, H.-P., 2012. Recent developments and future directions in Guillain-Barré syndrome. Journal Peripher Nerve System 17 (Suppl. 3), 57–70.

Meythaler, J.M., 1997. Rehabilitation of Guillain-Barré syndrome. Archives of Physical Medicine and Rehabilitation 78 (8), 872–879.

13

Monti Bragadin, M., Francini, L., Bellone, E., Grandis, M., Reni, L., Canneva, S., et al., 2015. Tinetti and Berg balance scales correlate with disability in hereditary peripheral neuropathies: a preliminary study. European Journal Physiology Rehabilition Medicine 51 (4), 423–427.

O'Connor, J., McCaughan, D., McDaid, C., Booth, A., Fayter, D., Rodriguez-Lopez, R., et al., 2016. Orthotic management of instability of the knee related to neuromuscular and central nervous system disorders: systematic review, qualitative study, survey and costing analysis. Health Technology Assess Winchester England 20 (55), 1–262.

Padua, L., Pazzaglia, C., Pareyson, D., Schenone, A., Aiello, A., Fabrizi, G.M., et al., 2016. Novel outcome measures for Charcot-Marie-Tooth disease: validation and reliability of the 6-min walk test and StepWatch(TM) Activity Monitor and identification of the walking features related to higher quality of life. European Journal Neurology 23 (8), 1343–1350.

Phillips, M., Radford, K., Wills, A., 2011. Ankle foot orthoses for people with Charcot Marie Tooth disease – views of users and orthotists on important aspects of use. Disability Rehabilitation Assited Technology 6 (6), 491–499.

Piscosquito, G., Reilly, M.M., Schenone, A., Fabrizi, G.M., Cavallaro, T., Santoro, L., et al., 2015. Responsiveness of clinical outcome measures in Charcot-Marie-Tooth disease. European Journal of Neurology 22 (12), 1556–1563.

Ramdharry, G.M., Carr, A., Laura, M., 2018. Polyneuropathies. In: Lennon, S., Ramdharry, G., Verheyden, G. (Eds.), Physical Management in Neurological Conditions, fourth ed, Elsevier, London, UK.

Ramdharry, G.M., Pollard, A.J., Marsden, J.F., Reilly, M.M., 2012a. Comparing gait performance of people with charcot-marie-tooth disease who do and do not wear ankle foot orthoses. Physiother Research International Journal Research Clinic Physics Theraputices 17 (4), 191–199.

Ramdharry, G.M., Thornhill, A., Mein, G., Reilly, M.M., Marsden, J.F., 2012b. Exploring the experience of fatigue in people with Charcot-Marie-Tooth disease. Neuromuscular Disorders NMD 22 (Suppl. 3), S208-S213.

Sackley, C., Disler, P.B., Turner-Stokes, L., Wade, D.T., Brittle, N., Hoppitt, T., 2009. Rehabilitation interventions for foot drop in neuromuscular disease. Cochrane Database Systems Review 3. CD003908.

Schwid, S.R., Thornton, C.A., Pandya, S., Manzur, K.L., Sanjak, M., Petrie, M.D., et al., 1999. Quantitative assessment of motor fatigue and strength in MS. Neurology 53 (4), 743–750.

Shumway-Cook, A., Horak, F.B., 1986. Assessing the influence of sensory interaction of balance. Suggestion from the field. Physical Therapy 66 (10), 1548–1550.

Simatos Arsenault, N., Vincent, P.-O., Yu, B.H.S., Bastien, R., Sweeney, A., 2016. Influence of exercise on patients with guillain-barré syndrome: a systematic review. Physiother Cancer 68 (4), 367–376.

van den Berg, B., Walgaard, C., Drenthen, J., Fokke, C., Jacobs, B.C., van Doorn, P.A., 2014. Guillain–Barré syndrome: pathogenesis, diagnosis, treatment and prognosis. National Review Neurology 10 (8), 469–482.

van Doorn, P.A., 2013. Diagnosis, treatment and prognosis of Guillain-Barré syndrome (GBS). Presse Medicale Paris Free 1983 42 (6 Pt 2), e193–e201.

Vanhoutte, E.K., Faber, C.G., van Nes, S.I., Jacobs, B.C., van Doorn, P.A., van Koningsveld, R., et al., 2012. Modifying the medical research council grading system through rasch analyses. Brain Journal Neurologial 135 (Pt 5), 1639–1649.

van Nes, S.I., Vanhoutte, E.K., Faber, C.G., Garssen, M., van Doorn, P.A., Merkies, I.S.J., 2009. Improving fatigue assessment in immune-mediated neuropathies: the modified Rasch-built fatigue severity scale. Journal Peripher Nervenarzte Systems 14 (4), 268–278.

van Nes, S.I., Vanhoutte, E.K., van Doorn, P.A., Hermans, M., Bakkers, M., Kuitwaard, K., et al., 2011. Rasch-built Overall Disability Scale (R-ODS) for immune-mediated peripheral neuropathies. Neurology 76 (4), 337–345.

Videler, A.J., Beelen, A., Nollet, F., 2008. Manual dexterity and related functional limitations in hereditary motor and sensory neuropathy. An explorative study. Disability and Rehabilitation 30 (8), 634–638.

Vucic, S., Kiernan, M.C., Cornblath, D.R., 2009. Guillain-Barré syndrome: an update. Journal Clinical Neuroscience Official Journal Neurosurg Society Australas 16 (6), 733–741.

Wakerley, B.R., Uncini, A., Yuki, N., Attarian, S., Barreira, A.A., Chan, Y.-C., et al., 2014. Guillain–Barré and Miller Fisher syndromes—new diagnostic classification. National Review Neurology 10 (9), 537–544.

Willison, H.J., Jacobs, B.C., van Doorn, P.A., 2016. Guillain-Barré syndrome. Lancet 388 (10045), 717–727.

13

List of abbreviations

A&E: Accident & Emergency
ABGs: Arterial blood gases
ABI: Acquired brain injury
AD: Autonomic dysreflexia
ADL: Activities of daily living
AFO: Ankle foot orthosis
AIDP: Acute inflammatory demyelinating polyradiculoneuropathy
AIS: American Spinal Injuries Association Impairment Scale
AMAN: Acute motor axonal neuropathy
AMSAN: Acute motor sensory axonal neuropathy
AS: Ashworth Scale
ASIA: American Spinal Injuries Association
ASIS: Anterior superior iliac spine
BAEP: Brainstem-auditory evoked potential
BBS: Berg Balance Scale
BoNT-A: Botulinum toxin - A
BOS: Base of support
BP: Blood pressure
BPPV: Benign paroxysmal positional vertigo
CAD: Cough assist device
CBF: Cerebral blood flow
CES: Cauda equina syndrome
CIDP: Chronic inflammatory demyelinating polyradiculoneuropathy
CIMT: Constraint-induced movement therapy
CIQ: Community Integration Questionnaire
CNS: Central nervous system
COG: Centre of gravity
CPP: Cerebral perfusion pressure
CPSP: Central poststroke pain
CSF: Cerebrospinal fluid
CT: Computed tomography
CTE: Chronic traumatic encephalopathy
CVA: Cerebrovascular accident
DADL: Domestic activities of daily living
DAI: Diffuse axonal injury
DC: Discharge
DMT: Disease-modifying therapy
DNA: Deoxyribonucleic acid
DVT: Deep venous thrombosis
EBP: Evidence-based practice

ECG: Electrocardiogram
EDH: Extradural haematoma
EEG: Electroencephalography
EMG-NMS: Electromyography-triggered neuromuscular electrostimulation
EP: Evoked potentials
FAC: Functional Ambulation Categories
FBC: Full blood count
FES: Functional electrical stimulation
FIM: Functional Independence Measure
FiO_2: The fraction of inspired oxygen
FLAIR: Fluid attenuation inversion recovery
FOG: Freezing of gait
FVC: Forced vital capacity
GBS: Guillain–Barré syndrome
GCS: Glasgow Coma Scale
GHJ: Glenohumeral joint
GOAT: Galveston Orientation and Amnesia Test
GOS: Glasgow Outcome Scale
HEP: Home exercise program
HH: Homonymous hemianopia
HO: Heterotropic ossification
HOAC: Hypothesis-Oriented Algorithms for Clinicians
HPC: History of the present condition or complaint
IC: Initial contact
ICF: International Classification of Functioning, Disability and Health
ICP: Intracranial pressure
ICU: Intensive care unit
IPPB: Intermittent positive pressure breathing
ISCoS: International Spinal Cord Injury Society
ISNCSCI: International Standard Neurological Classification of Spinal Cord Injury
IVIg: Intravenous immunoglobulin
LACI: Lacunar infarct
LE: Lower extremity
LL: Lower limb
LMN: Lower motor neurone
LOC: Loss of consciousness
LP: Lumbar puncture
LR: Loading response

LVR: Lung volume recruitment
MAC: Manual assisted cough
MAP: Mean arterial pressure
MASCIP: Multidisciplinary Association of Spinal Cord Injury Professionals
MAS: Modified Ashworth Scale
MCS: Minimally conscious state
MDT: Multidisciplinary team
MELAS: Mitochondrial encephalopathy lactic acid and stroke
MERRF: Myoclonus epilepsy and ragged red fibres
MFS: Miller–Fisher syndrome
MHI: Manual hyperinflation
MIC: Maximal insufflation capacity
MIE: Mechanical insufflation and exsufflation
MMT: Manual muscle testing
MRC: Medical research council
MRI: Magnetic resonance imaging
MS: Multiple sclerosis
MST: Midstance
NCGS: National Clinical Guidelines for Stroke
NCS: Nerve conduction study
NHNN: National Hospital for Neurology & Neurosurgery
NHS: National Health Service
NICE: National Institute of Health and Care Excellence
NIHSS: National Institute of Health Stroke Scale
NIV: Noninvasive ventilation
NMS: Neuromuscular stimulation
OCSP: Oxford Community Stroke Project
OT: Occupational therapy
$PaCO_2$: Partial pressure of arterial carbon dioxide
PaO_2: Partial pressure of arterial oxygen
PACI: Partial anterior circulation infarct
PADL: Personal activities of daily living
PCF: Peak cough flow
PCR: Polymerase chain reaction
PEEP: Peak end expiratory pressure
PEFR: Peak expiratory flow rate
pH: Potential of hydrogen
POCI: Posterior circulation infarct
POMR: Problem-oriented medical record
PRE: Progressive resisted exercise
PS: Preswing
PTA: Posttraumatic amnesia
PVS: Persistent vegetative state

RAMP: Recovery, adaptation, maintenance, prevention
RCCs: Respiratory control centres
RCTs: Randomised controlled trials
REM: Rapid eye movement
ROM: Range of movement
RR: Respiratory rate
rt-PA: Recombinant tissue plasminogen activator
RUJ: Radioulnar joint
SCI: Spinal cord injury
SCIM: Spinal cord independence measure
SDH: Subdural haematoma
SH: Social history
SIGN: Scottish Intercollegiate Guidelines Network
SMART: Specific, measurable, achievable/ambitious, relevant, timed
SOAP: Subjective, objective, assessment, plan
SpO_2: Oxygen saturation
SSEP: Somatosensory evoked potentials
STREAM: Stroke Rehabilitation Assessment of Movement
SUTC: Stroke Unit Trialists Collaboration
TACI: Total anterior circulation infarct
TBI: Traumatic brain injury
TIA: Transient ischaemic attack
TILE: Task, Individual, Load, Environment
TMS: Transcranial magnetic stimulation
TOAST: Trial of Org 10172 in Acute Stroke Treatment
TST: Terminal stance
UK: United Kingdom
UL: Upper limb
UMN: Upper motor neurone
UMNS: Upper motor neurone syndrome
UN: Unilateral neglect
UTI: Urinary tract infection
UWS: Unresponsive wakefulness syndrome
VC: Vital capacity
VEP: Visual evoked potentials
VHI: Ventilator hyperinflation
VOR: Vestibular ocular reflex
VR: Vestibular rehabilitation
VS: Vegetative state
WCPT: World Confederation for Physical Therapy
WHO: World Health Organization
WT: Weight transference

Note: Page numbers followed by *f* indicate figures, *t* indicate tables, and *b* indicate boxes.